ADVANCE PRAISE F [barcode]
BE HEALTHY ~~ ~~~~ ~~~~

"I have practiced holistic medicine for over 30 years. I can testify that Jane Falke walks her talk. She is the healthiest 71 year old I have ever had the pleasure of having as a patient. She looks like an attractive, fit and active '50 something.' Jane is her own best advertisement and highest credential. I will recommend Eat Healthy. Be Healthy at Any Age. *to all my patients."*
~ Dr. John H. Maher, board certified in clinical nutrition and integrative medicine, postgraduate faculty in anti-aging medicine www.valleycenterholistic.com, Valley Center, CA

"Eat Healthy. Be Healthy at Any Age. IS UNIQUE, and it will be the last healthy eating book you'll need. You're going to love understanding how YOU can be in control of how you feel. People who look at Jane Falke are always amazed. She looks 20 years younger than her age and she is radiantly healthy. As Jane says, 'What we eat is the problem AND the solution.' This means you have the power to be as healthy and young as you want to be. Avoid suffering and the side effects of drugs. Buy this book and find out how to make health your wealth."
~ Doris Helge, Ph.D. and author of *Transforming Pain into Power* and other best-sellers

"Good health starts with good choices, and Eat Healthy. Be Healthy at Any Age. *is like an encyclopedia on healthy choices like nothing I have read in 20 years in the health care profession. In a simple to read and understand style, 'Dr.' Jane shows how it can be both fun and easy to take back control of your personal health with a teaspoon of responsibility, understanding and perseverance."*
~ Dr. Mark Elliott, DC Performance Chiropractic Center / Spine Decompression Center, Vista, CA

"In the last three decades I've read dozens of books on health and nutrition. Out of all of them, Eat Healthy. Be Healthy at Any Age. *by Jane Falke is by far one of the best. Not only does the author share her big WHY as to what motivated her to learn, study and become an expert at alkaline eating, her writing is such that it is very engaging and easy to follow.*

The information provided is insightful, informative and in many ways shocking. No wonder we are such an unhealthy culture.

Jane Falke offers detail as to how we got here and what to do to get on the road to optimal health as quickly as possible.

If you're looking for the next magic pill to get you healthy, this book is not for you. If you're looking for solid information based on real science, you will love this book.

Eat Healthy. Be Healthy at Any Age. *is a great read for someone new to studying healthy eating to those who have studied virtually every diet and eating regime known to mankind."*
~ Kathleen Gage, marketing and online strategist
www.kathleengage.com

"I know that my commitment to making the world a better place begins as an inside job. It starts within each of us. Thank you for showing us how to be the best we can be with Eat Healthy. Be Healthy at Any Age.*"*
~ Karyn Garvin, The Divine Dog Trainer, author
of *Dogs Do Go to Heaven.*
www.DogTrainingEquipment.com

"Jane Falke has written a clear, fact filled picture of nutritional information that will knock your socks off. I plan on using Eat Healthy. Be Healthy at Any Age. *to improve my health and well-being. I liked her examples and positive presentation on a subject that is important for us all. I am excited to jump into a new level of health care for myself!"*
~ Eva Roza, President, Roza Real Estate Loans, Inc., San Francisco, CA

"I went to Jane because I was overweight, listless and had no energy, plus I was diagnosed with breast cancer. I followed the plan Jane teaches in Eat Healthy. Be Heathly at Any Age. *and lost 15 lbs.! Now my energy level is at 100%, and my eating habits have totally changed for the better. I am so excited with my results."*
~ Laurie Elliott, Pauma Valley, CA

"Jane Falke's Eat Healthy. Be Healthy at Any Age. *provides the techniques to change your health by changing what you eat. I loved the ideas that 'nutritious food is like premium gas' and that you can 'eat to live' rather than 'live to eat.' This book is clear and easy to understand. I know I can improve my health and slow down the aging process by following the information in this book."*
~ JoAnne Skelly, Associate Professor, University of Nevada, Reno; Extension Educator, Cooperative Extension, Reno, NV

"Jane Falke's nutritional passion and knowledge is shared in this detailed book, Eat Healthy. Be Healthy at Any Age. *Concisely written and practical, Jane makes it easy for you to eat healthy and be healthy."*
~ Dr. Debra Asakura, DC, www.AdvancedSpineandJointCare.com, Vista, CA

"From the first paragraph when Jane invited me to go on a journey with her to experience life without pain or suffering I couldn't stop reading. As a registered nurse I have cared for people who made themselves sick because of unhealthy eating. I wish I could have shared this book with them. My personal story found me filling my body with empty calories and with what I learned from Jane I am now enjoying a healthy life. Jane offers knowledge and a process that is couched in caring, and her support is infused into each word and step to health. Jane truly is on the journey with you. This is an important life-saving book. Don't wait to read and use it."

~ Suzanne Ward, MA, MN, RN, CNOR (e), GC-C

Eat Healthy.
Be Healthy
at Any Age.

Discover Why Food
Is the Problem
as Well as the Solution

By Jane Falke, M.S.

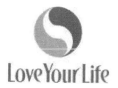

Love Your Life

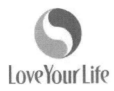

Love Your Life Publishing
www.loveyourlifepublishing.com
ISBN: 978-1-934509-66-1
Library of Congress Control Number: 2012954585
Printed in the United States of America
First Printing 2013
Cover design: www.Cyanotype.ca
Editing by Gwen Hoffnagle

Disclaimer:

Any advice regarding aspects of physical, mental, or emotional health is not meant to be a replacement or substitution for medical advice from a licensed physician or mental health professional. Always consult a health care professional if you have any issues with your health. The Author will not be held liable for any advice, suggestions, or opinions given in any session, article, or book.

CONTENTS

Eat Healthy. Be Healthy at Any Age.

Introduction

Congratulations for making the decision to be healthy. There are obviously many benefits to good health. The most important benefit is that *you can have a life without suffering or pain.*

When we are sick, we want to get rid of the illness – fast. We not only want to feel better, we want our lives to get back to normal. We go to the doctor or take medications or nutritional supplements thinking one of these efforts will solve our problem, and we may be able to relieve our symptoms. But what about the cause of the illness? Are we addressing the cause with such treatments? When we feel better, we go back to living, eating, and thinking in the same old ways – aches, pains, and illnesses again creep into our lives. So in the end we are not truly mended.

Hippocrates, known as the Father of Medicine, was a Greek physician who lived in the third and fourth centuries BC. He believed the body has the power to heal itself with a healthy diet, rest, and cleanliness. He is often quoted as saying, "Let food be thy medicine and medicine be thy food." Most of our medical professionals believe that drugs, along with certain procedures and therapies, are the proper approach to healing. But the body is the real healer. Many drugs and procedures help with some health issues, but at the high cost of adding toxins to the body. Toxins can challenge the parts of the body not being targeted for healing and cause additional problems with which the body must deal. Giving the body what it needs to heal itself is a natural approach. Why have we removed ourselves from Hippocrates's method? Could the answer be in the kind of food we eat?

Eat Healthy. Be Healthy at Any Age.

Hippocrates's natural approach resonates with me. The American diet has changed, and new diseases are on the increase. More and more manufactured products are available at food markets. Because our lives are so fast-paced, many of us do not take the time to prepare healthy meals. We buy meals already prepared, as pre-packaged convenience meals, canned or frozen foods, or at fast-food establishments. With this change in diet comes a change in our health.

My daughter was diagnosed with type I diabetes. She controls it with insulin injections and diet. I had to learn how to care for her, and it was a quite a learning experience. "Nutrition? What is that?" I had to learn how to balance my daughter's diet through the proper amounts of proteins, carbohydrates, and fats at every meal. My daughter's illness sparked my interest in eating healthy food to control disease and improve health.

In the early 1990s, I began seriously studying nutrition when my husband was diagnosed with cancer. It was too late for him to change his habits. The disease metastasized throughout his small intestines. His diet was questionable, but it was his choice to eat what he ate. He was what we call a meat and potatoes man. He used to say, "My doctor said I was allergic to vegetables. I shouldn't eat them." Within six months after diagnosis, he passed away.

My mother was diagnosed with Alzheimer's disease. Over a twelve-year period I watched her slowly crumble from a happy adult to a child. She could no longer take care of her simplest needs. Her diet was high in proteins, refined carbohydrates, sugar, and fats.

It is heartbreaking to see loved ones suffer with such pain. Medical doctors did not have a clue as to what actually caused these diseases. Nor could their advanced technologies cure them. From these experiences I gained the conviction that we are not born on this planet to suffer and die an early death. I decided to search for the root causes of disease to help change the course of illnesses. I began studying food and nutrition as solutions to poor health.

I have seen much suffering, depression, and signs of diseases while coaching clients to balance their nutrition through diet and through live and dry blood analysis. It saddens me that disease and suffering is so widespread when a simple, natural way of eating can sustain our health.

With proper knowledge and planning, you can make changes to overcome many health challenges. Maintaining good health is so important. *Eat Healthy. Be Healthy at Any Age* provides the understanding of how food likely causes health problems, and how healthy eating is an achievable solution.

Part I of this book presents easy-to-understand facts about how to balance your intake of nutrition from food. I discuss the importance of ingesting proper nutrients through healthy foods and appropriate supplements. Nutrients continually repair the body and keep it healthy. You will also learn which foods are good for your health and which foods are not.

Part II includes my programs, an easy-to-follow plan for removing toxins from the body, the foundation and building blocks of good health, and suggested menu plans. You will learn how whole natural foods help the body continually heal and repair itself naturally without drugs. These healthy-eating programs can help you succeed with your health goals.

And in Part III are the delicious, easy-to-prepare recipes for the programs and to keep you on the path to good health.

Eat Healthy. Be Healthy at Any Age.

I wrote *Eat Healthy. Be Healthy at Any Age* so you can benefit from my work and experiences. All I ask is that you keep an open mind and read the book all the way through before starting the programs or deciding whether this dietary change is for you.

Good health is a journey, and the most important natural resource for your well-being. The biggest benefits from healthy eating are a change in your health and a change in your appearance. How about giving your body the gift of vibrant health!

Chapter 1
My Story of Radiant Health

I didn't grow up in a family that knew about eating food for good health. We ate because we were hungry. I ate what was put on my plate, except the vegetables. But my father wouldn't let me leave the dinner table unless I finished the food on my plate. If I didn't, he fed it to me. I cried and cried while he shoveled the vegetables into my mouth. Canned vegetables? Dreadful!

During my teen years, I ate more and more canned foods and acquired enough of a taste for those dreadful vegetables to eat them, though I still didn't like them. It was rare to be served fresh vegetables at my house. But when I was at my grandmother's house for dinner, she served many fresh vegetables. She had a garden in her back yard, and we used to go into the garden and pick vegetables for dinner. Those vegetables had great flavor and texture. All the grandchildren and great grandchildren used to walk into my grandmother's house, give her a kiss, and open the refrigerator to see what there was to eat. We loved Nona's cooking. It was fresh. She never used canned or packaged foods.

Eat Healthy. Be Healthy at Any Age.

After I was married, I had to learn how to cook. I used to call my mother and grandmother every day to find out how to make dinner. (I never thought about buying a cookbook.) I mostly used my grandmother's suggestions. Yes, you guessed why – they were fresh and tasted so much better. I became very good at preparing fresh meals, but they included what everyone was eating at that time: a large portion of meat cooked in butter, margarine, or vegetable oil, potatoes or rice with perhaps gravy or sauce, and a side of vegetables slathered with butter or margarine. This is what I knew then.

Today my meal plate looks very different. Why did I change my food choices over time? Because I learned more about how food relates to health. It started when my daughter was diagnosed with type I diabetes. I learned there was a relationship between controlling diabetes and proper diet. Later I realized my husband wasn't eating a balanced diet, and therefore wasn't getting the proper nutrients to help with any kind of healing. He died an early death without realizing his dreams.

When my mother died from Alzheimer's disease, it put me over the top in regard to healthy eating. After her passing, I cleaned out her house. Her pantry was filled with old cans of food. The freezer was packed with frozen items that had been there for years. The herbs and spices were antiques. I was shocked, and it triggered a burning desire to find out why some people have certain diseases while others do not, and what causes disease in general.

Thus began my quest to find healthy options to aging and death by disease. I tested many diets on myself to experience the results, not only in my appearance and my health, but in my energy level as well. The high-protein, high-fat, low-carbohydrate diet was constipating. Counting calories was annoying. Keeping track of points didn't provide a balanced diet. Eating a high-starch diet made me gain weight. Foods from cans and packages provided by various diet companies were missing the fresh flavors I love, and I wondered what else was missing! Even the so-called "health plans" I was learning about through my nutrition studies were questionable.

But when I started eating plant-based, whole foods, I started feeling healthy. You may have read about the suitability of different diets to different blood types, and you might be thinking that I just have the type of blood that's compatible with plant-based foods. You might be thinking, "I'm a hunter-gatherer. I require protein." I address this subject in the coming chapters.

I received my certification as a yoga teacher in 1991, and that was when I seriously began transitioning to a plant-based diet. I received my master's degree in holistic nutrition and training in live and dry blood analysis in 2010. Blood analysis offers my clients a visual way to see the health of their blood. Often this is motivation enough to change their food choices in order to change their health.

At this writing I am seventy-one years young. I meditate and practice yoga regularly. I follow the health program in this book and regard myself as healthy in spite of all the pollution in our world. I do face challenges from time to time, and consider these wake-up calls that something I'm doing isn't working and I need to make a change. I'm certain this happens to you, too, and I know you would rather have good health than a challenge. Here's to your health.

Isn't it time to do all you can to maintain your health through the years you have left?

Chapter 2
Change Your Health by Changing Your Eating

Most people resist change because they are fearful and don't know what the change will bring them. But remaining in the status quo will only give you what you have right now. Are you satisfied with your life the way it is now? Probably not, since you are reading this book.

Discomfort is a motivating factor in our lives that usually brings about change. Humans are meant to experience life rather than stay in the same place; experiences are what make you grow. Growth leads to more learning experiences and further change and growth. This is the way life is meant to be.

And so it is with your health. If you want to change a health condition, improve your health, or slow down aging, you will have to change the way you eat and the way you think about food. The major diseases we die from – heart disease, stroke, and some cancers – are caused by poor nutrition and poor eating habits. Many health conditions can be improved or controlled through balanced nutrition and healthy food choices.

There are many diets that are thought to be healthy. If you are eating mostly or exclusively plant-based foods, you are on the right track. Eating animals that eat an unnatural diet; live in crowded, feces-filled facilties; and consume chemically laden, processed foods contributes to unhealthy conditions and disease in our society.

If you have low energy, fatigue, poor digestion, excess weight, unclear thinking, diarrhea, constipation, skin rashes, arthritis, osteoporosis, or heart disease (I could go on, but I think you get the point), you have a nutritionally controllable health condition. If you don't change the way you eat, conditions can worsen as time goes on.

Illnesses like the ones listed above start with a disturbance or irritation in the body. You usually don't notice it because the disturbance is internal. It can harm the internal environment of the body by impacting the quality of your cells. Cells make up your blood and every part of your body. When cells are sick, you are sick. This is the cycle of imbalance, and poorer and poorer health results if you don't stop the cycle. It's time to take control of what goes into your mouth, eliminate chronic conditions, and be healthy!

The control you have over your life lies in the choices and decisions you make. To have control over your health means making the right choices about what you eat and how you eat. Choosing healthy, whole natural foods keeps your cells alive and functioning and provides your body with a nutritious, balanced diet.

One problem with the Western diet has to do with taste. People want to eat what they are familiar with or identify as tasting good. But many items we eat are not real food; they are laced with added chemicals. Even though all food is made up of chemicals, it's the chemicals added by manufacturers that are the problem. Just look at the ingredients lists on packaged foods. What ends up in a bottle of salad dressing or a box of cereal may not be what nature provides. It is usually a mixture of chemicals that our taste buds have become familiar with, and we say, "This tastes good."

Did you know there is a flavor industry? Flavorists help enhance the taste of foods. They copy natural flavors using synthetic chemicals. One Swiss company, Gevaudan, is a multi-national company that mimics Mother Nature's molecules to create an equal flavor. Food manufacturing companies and restaurants buy these flavors and add them to their foods as "natural flavors." These "natural flavors" are not food; they are added chemicals. These chemical flavors provide a pleasurable taste experience, but they are stimulating and addicting so that you will keep buying them. That's how artificial flavors and "natural flavors" lead to overconsumption.[1]

Processed foods contain stabilizers along with the sugar, salt, refined grains, refined oils, chemical additives, and preservatives. The purpose of stabilizers is to improve the taste, texture, and shelf life. One common stabilizer is monosodium glutamate (MSG) – the "flavor enhancer." MSG has many alliases. "Natural flavors" are one of many ingredients that can convert to MSG during processing.[2] Food manufacturers' practice of using various names in ingredients lists is a way to disguise such chemical additives.

In their book, *The Slow Poisoning of America*, John and T. Michelle Erb report that MSG in food makes us eat more of a product and choose it over one that doesn't have MSG because it has addictive qualities.[3] MSG is not regulated by any government agency. It can be added to foods in any amount. It does enhance flavor, but also enhances your addiction to those foods.

6

The Western diet includes so many fast foods and processed foods that we have lost our taste for what nature provides from the garden. We have grown so accustomed to eating fatty, salty, sugary, refined carbohydrates and chemical-laden foods that our taste buds have changed, and our waistlines and our health have changed right along with them.

Our taste buds can change back to liking natural foods just as easily as they adapted to chemical additives. We can make them adapt to real food by cleansing the body of waste, breaking destructive eating habits that disturb or irritate the cells in our bodies, and providing our bodies with foods that make healthy cells. If you need help changing destructive habits, my guided meditation can help. Download it at www.janefalke. com/changing-your-habit-patterns.

The benefits of whole natural foods are many. First and foremost is healthy blood. If you have healthy blood, you have good health in your body. Here are just a few more benefits of eating the balanced nutrition of whole foods:

- Alive and vibrant internal drive
- A pain-free body
- High energy levels to support what you want to do in life
- Soft, young-looking, blemish-free skin
- Slower aging so you can live longer
- A lean and trim body, as nature intended
- Taste buds that return to normal so you can enjoy natural food again
- Uncongested head and nasal passages
- Youthful appearance
- Clear thinking
- Better concentration
- No more sugar cravings

Eat Healthy. Be Healthy at Any Age.

- Lower LDL (bad) cholesterol and total cholesterol
- Higher HDL (good) cholesterol
- Regular bowel movements
- Less likelihood of suffering or dying from a disease

And, most of all, *you will save money* on doctor bills, prescriptions, and other therapies because you will not have chronic diseases that need medical atttention. You will also save money on nutritional supplements, as healthy, whole natural foods provide your body with the nutrients it needs. This should be motivation enough to do something about your health and do it now, before health conditions show up or worsen.

Thomas Edison said, "The doctor of the future will give no medicine, but will interest his patients in the care of the human frame, in diet, and in the cause and prevention of disease." There are a small number of doctors who educate their patients about diet. Does your doctor give you advice about disease prevention and diet? If not, you can educate yourself by reading this book.

Because you are reading *Eat Healthy. Be Healthy at Any Age.*, there must be a message here for you. All I ask is that you remain open to the information and give it a try. Even four weeks on The Maintenance Program will prove to you that changes are happening in your health and in your body. It is time for a change. You can have better health in a few weeks and vibrant health in a few months. All you have to do is apply the programs in this book.

Chapter 3
Who Controls Our Food?

Genetically Engineered or Modified Foods

Companies create foods that resist pests so they can grow more food, patent the modified seeds, and control the food supply throughout the world. In their book, *Genetically Engineered Food: A Self-Defense Guide for Consumers,* authors Ronnie Cummins and Ben Lilliston describe *genetic engineering* as altering genetic blueprints of living organisms by introducing them into another host organism to create a new, genetically engineered organism.[1]

Here are some concerns about this practice from Wikipedia:[2]

- DNA is changed
- Unknown long-term health effects
- Environmental safety
- Labeling and consumer choice
- Ethics
- Food security
- Environmental conservation
- Potential disruption or even possible destruction of the food chain
- Potential or actual health or ecological disaster

Eat Healthy. Be Healthy at Any Age.

The Organic Consumers Association says that most genetically engineered (GE) foods are not available in supermarkets as whole foods. Rather, they come to us as processed foods. Genetically engineered crops – primarily corn, canola, and soy – are added to animal feed and used as ingredients in processed foods. It is estimated that at least 60 percent of processed foods on the market currently contain ingredients derived from genetically engineered soybeans.[3]

Cummins and Lilliston say additives in processed foods are examples of genetically modified (GM) products, such as:

- Dextrose, fructose, maltose, and sucrose are in sweet products like desserts and soft drinks.
- Aspartame is added to children's vitamins; medicines; chewing gum; many low-fat products such as jelly, jam, sodas, and yogurt; and some candy.
- Maltodextrin is used as filler for gravy mixes and flavored chips.
- Xanthan gum is used as a thickener in ice cream, salad dressing, and confectionery products.
- Yeasts and enzymes are used to produce cheese to make an unnatural product.[4]

The Institute for Responsible Technology has produced a shopping guide called Non-GMO Shopping Tips: How to Avoid Foods Made with Genetically Modified Organisms. Tip #1: Buy organic. Certified organic products cannot intentionally include any GM ingredients. Buy products labeled "100% organic," "Organic," or "Made with organic ingredients." You can be doubly sure if the product also has a "Non-GMO Project Verified" seal. You can download a complete list of hidden food sources by going to www. NonGMOShoppingGuide.com. The list of such products is a long one. Rest assured, if you buy processed and packaged foods, and not 100 percent organic, you are buying and eating GM foods.

In his book *Seeds of Deception: Exposing Industry and Government Lies about the Safety of the Genetically Engineered Foods You're Eating,* Jeffrey Smith states, "The easiest ways to avoid these are to either buy products listed as organic or non-GMO, or prepare your own foods from basic, unprocessed ingredients." (pp. 243, 244) (In my opinion, Jeffrey Smith is the guru of knowledge about GMO foods.)

Arran Stephens wrote the preface for *Seeds of Deception,* in which he says this about GM foods: "We are now in the middle of the largest feeding experiment in history and we human beings are the guinea pigs."[5]

Also in *Seeds of Deception,* Jeffery Smith cites a report from the *Washington Post:* Rodents usually munch on tomatoes but turned their noses up at GM FlavrSavr tomatoes. Rats were eventually force-fed the GM tomatoes through gastric tubes. Several developed stomach lesions; seven of forty died within two weeks. The tomato was approved for human consumption.[6]

The animals we eat consume GM foods as part of their food supply; corn and soy are staples in their diets, and they assimilate these gene alterations into their bodies. When we eat animal products, genetic mutations become part of us. We have no idea what will happen to our species as generations go by as a result of altered DNA. And our children and unborn children are the most vulnerable to the potential effects of eating these foods.

When given a choice between conventionally grown products and genetically modified products, feedlot animals choose conventionally grown feed over GM feed. GM foods are pest resistant. Does it make sense that pests and rodents do not eat genetically modified foods, but humans do?

Ingredients labels are not required to specify whether ingredients are genetically engineered, so you can't tell whether you're eating these products unless the label specifically says you are not. Soy, corn, cotton seed, and canola ingredients in packaged and processed foods are more than likely genetically engineered.

Organically Grown Food

I am sure you have heard about some of the benefits of organic foods, but you may be discouraged from buying them because they're expensive, or you think you can buy conventionally grown foods and wash off the pesticides. Organically grown food is usually more expensive for several reasons:

- The government does not subsidize organic farmers as it does large agribusiness.
- There are extra costs involved in following the strict guidelines required to claim that a food is organic and to carry the organic seal. Essentially we have to pay more for what is *not* in our food – pesticides, herbicides, antibiotics, and hormones – than for foods not produced with these extra toxins.
- It is more labor-intensive to produce organic food, further increasing production costs.

However, demand makes prices go down. And the higher cost justifies the healthy benefits of eating food grown organically.

Organic describes a way of growing agricultural products using methods that encourage soil and water preservation and reduce toxic waste. Organic farmers employ practices such as crop rotation and mulching instead of using chemical herbicides. They use natural fertilizers instead of chemically produced fertilizers to improve soil for ideal plant growth and nutrition. They use beneficial insects instead of insecticides to reduce pests and disease.[7] Organically grown plants include vegetables, fruits, nuts, seeds, legumes, and grains, and "organic" also refers to animal products and by-products (such as cheese and eggs) from animals that eat organic feed.

Much of the food industry produces conventionally grown foods. The industry looks for ways to yield more food and keep it fresh longer. Herbicides, insecticides, and fungicides are applied to crops and soil to kill the weeds, pests, and fungi that destroy crops. These poisons go into the ground, the roots of the plants absorb them, and in turn their cells absorb them while the plants are growing. More plants grow larger, but at a price to our health. You cannot wash these poisons off, and they eventually become the meal on your plate.

The food industry also has ways to keep food from rotting in storage and on the shelves at grocery stores. They use irradiation – exposing food to gamma rays – to keep the food from spoiling. The food does last longer, but the radiation not only keeps bacteria from eating the food, it also kills the natural enzymes in food. Enzymes are important because they allow food to start digestion when you eat it.

When you eat foods grown with genetically altered seed, sprayed with chemicals, and shot with gamma rays, toxic buildup in your body rises while nutrition in your food has been reduced. Hormones added to animal feed make animals grow faster. Antibiotics added to animal feed stave off disease. Your body needs nutrients to

Eat Healthy. Be Healthy at Any Age.

survive, not these added chemicals and drugs. Your body can become more toxic from eating chemically treated animals and conventionally grown foods.

Synthetic chemicals seep into our soil and run off into our waterways, eventually harming wildlife and our environment. Millions of gallons of these chemicals are used on our food each year, and they have an influence on our health, just as wildlife down soil and downstream from crops suffers health consequences. Food allergies, infertility, birth defects, neurological disorders, cancer, and heart disease are just some of the health disorders that occur due to toxic chemical exposure.

In the United States, ingredients labels on packaged foods are not required to state whether a product contains genetically engineered ingredients. Even many restaurants buy processed products to prepare their meals. Genetically altered foods are everywhere in our food supply. We must be cautious what and where we eat.

Packaged food labels show whether a product contains organically grown ingredients. The Food and Drug Administration allows a "USDA Organic" symbol on organic products. Products labeled "100% organic" must contain at least 95 percent organically grown products. Products that are below 70 percent organically produced can only list their organic ingredients on the ingredients label.

Stickers on fruits and vegetables have numbers on them. When the number has five digits, and the first number is nine (such as 95381), that item has been organically grown. When the number has four digits, and the first number is three or four (such as 4321 or 3221), that item has been conventionally grown. When the number has five digits, and the first number is eight, that item has been genetically modified. But you may never see a number beginning with eight, as there is no regulation for labeling genetically engineered food. The manufacturers of GM seeds do not want you to know you are eating them. They do not use stickers to identify GM foods.

The Environmental Working Group analyzed pesticide residue test data from the US Department of Agriculture and the Food and Drug Administration to come up with rankings for the following popular fresh produce items. Below are the "dirty dozen."[8] *(Lower numbers equal more pesticides.)*

1. Apples

2. Celery

3. Strawberries

4. Peaches

5. Spinach

6. Nectarines – imported

7. Grapes – imported

8. Sweet bell peppers

9. Potatoes

10. Blueberries - domestic

11. Lettuce

12. Kale/collard greens

Organic plant foods supply your body with pure oxygen and naturally filtered water, and they are great sources of the vitamins, minerals, and enzymes that keep you healthy. This is why organic food is considered high-quality food. To keep yourself healthy, consider buying and eating fresh food grown organically.

Eat Healthy. Be Healthy at Any Age.

The Forces behind Our Food

We are constantly bombarded with marketing and advertising on TV, on the street, at stores, and in restaurants. Pictures of food are in our sight wherever we go. Temptation is around every corner, making it easy to eat low-priced, low-quality food anytime. Convenience is tempting.

With our fast-paced lives, making time to plan and prepare healthy meals can be a challenge, and this is where the problem lies. We end up eating refined foods with low to no nutrient value; high in sugar, salt, and bad fats; and loaded with chemical additives. These additives are addictive and cause food cravings. You have satisfied your hunger, but you are hungry again in a few short hours. Eating foods depleted of nutrients leads to malnutrition. You eat more, but actually starve your body of nutrients, so the cycle of eating starts all over again. Your body needs nutrients and signals you to eat. You end up paying for more food, not only with your money, but also with your waistline and your health.

In the documentary movie, *Super-Size Me*, Morgan Spurlock solves the obesity epidemic while interviewing experts and putting his own body through a test – the "McDonald's only" diet – for thirty days straight. The movie discusses corporate responsibility, nutritional education, and school lunch programs, and how we as a nation are eating ourselves to death.[9]

Morgan wanted to see what would happen to his health during this month-long diet. The rules were: 1) He had to eat three meals a day at McDonald's. 2) If asked "Do you want to supersize?" he had to say yes. 3) He had to eat everything on the menu during the thirty days. 4) If McDonald's did not sell it, he could not eat it.

Spurlock documented the condition of his health before, during, and after his month-long eating plan. He was tested by a cardiologist, a gastroenterologist, and a general practitioner. He saw a dietician and an exercise physiologist. His results showed he was in good shape, at a good weight, and in good health before he embarked on the diet.

These were the consequences:

- After 5 days – gained 5 percent of body weight, felt depressed, felt pressure in his chest, and felt exhausted.
- After 12 days – gained 17 pounds.
- After 18 days – headaches, felt bad, and cholesterol went from 165 to 225.
- After 21 days – could not breathe, felt hot, and had heart palpations. Doctors advised him to stop the diet because his liver was failing.
- After 30 days – gained 24 ½ pounds, liver turned to fat, cholesterol jumped up 65 points, body fat went from 11 percent to 18 percent, depressed and exhausted most of the time, mood changes, sex "0." He craved food more when he ate it and had headaches when he did not eat it. He had consumed 30 pounds of sugar and 12 pounds of fat.

Think about how often you eat fast food during a thirty-day period. Maybe you're wondering why you feel badly and are hungry all the time. As you eat more of such food, you want more. Is it any wonder that we are an overweight and obese nation? Morgan's experience could be what you are experiencing. Fast food is addicting. The only way to change your health is to make better choices about what and where you eat.

Nutrition Action magazine interviewed Marion Nestle, author of *Food Politics: How the Food Industry*

Eat Healthy. Be Healthy at Any Age.

Influences Nutrition and Health, about how the food industry influences what we eat. This is what came out of the interview:

The food industry is a commanding influence behind our food choices. Its purpose is to make money selling its products. Its publically traded companies not only have to make sales, they have to increase their profits every quarter. They do it in several ways:

- Marketing and advertising campaigns. They advertise on television during certain times that will benefit their sales. Children's programs are very profitable.
- Putting their products in vending machines at schools, sports facilities, and airports.
- Adding something to their product consumers think is healthy.
- Paying supermarkets to place their products at eye level, on aisle-end displays, and near registers.

Do you think the government will protect you from the food companies and their products? Every food company has a lobbyist working for them who is responsible for keeping their products in good standing with government agencies.[10] Their products remain in the food supply even though they may not be healthy for us.

Dr. T. Colin Campbell, in his book *The China Study: Startling Implications for Diet, Weight Loss and Long-term Health, says,* "There are powerful, influential, and enormously wealthy industries that stand to lose a vast amount of money if Americans start shifting to a plant-based diet. Their financial health depends on controlling what the public knows about nutrition and health."[11]

Control over government regulations does not only apply to the food industry. Control comes from pharmaceutical companies as well. Pharmaceutical companies have to be profitable. They financially support and promote their drugs in medical schools. They supply drug samples and incentives to doctors so doctors will prescribe their drugs to patients. It is reported that consumers pay more for their "medicine" in the US than in any other country in the world. Does that make you feel better?

Drugs are meant to improve your health. The added "benefit" is that you can acquire side effects from them. Taking certain prescribed medications over a long period of time can cause allergies, headaches, and organ failure.

How Can You Deal with These Influences?

If you are overweight, obese, or have been diagnosed with insulin resistance, metabolic syndrome, prediabetes, or type II diabetes, it is time to look at what and where you are eating. The only way to stop the vicious cycle of poor health and questionable eating habits is to stop eating what you are eating right now. It isn't working!

Many people take excellent care of their homes, gardens, and automobiles; why not spend at least as much effort caring for your body and your health? Waiting for something to happen to you before making changes can mean being too late. Committing to your health is the best start for change. Do it NOW!

PART I:
Sustaining Health with Balanced Nutrition

When your body is assimilating high-quality nutrients every day, that is ideal nutrition. This keeps you functioning well, mentally and physically, by increasing your energy and protecting you from disease. Denying your body ideal nutrition can cause irreparable damage and lead to chronic disease and early death. This is why knowledge about what you eat is so important in maintaining good health.

Food is fuel for the body. Nutritious food is like premium gas. Deficient food is like putting oil in your gas tank and expecting your car to perform as usual. Whole, natural foods provide premium gas: absorbable nutrients. Processed and refined foods are the oil: deficient in nutrients.

Our reasons for eating are many:

- it is a social event with friends and family
- to soothe our emotional swings
- it looks and tastes good and the smell triggers something in our minds and mouths to want it
- because of food addictions and food cravings
- because the food industry makes eating so inviting

We eat when we want to instead of when we are hungry. We are living to eat, not eating to live.

Nutrients gained through what you eat and drink are essential for life. They consist of macronutrients and micronutrients. *Macronutrients* are carbohydrates, fats, and proteins. *Micronutrients* are vitamins, minerals, antioxidants, and phytonutrients. When you eat macronutrients, you absorb and assimilate the micronutrients in them. This is what keeps your body functioning at its best, and it's the way we were intended to obtain our nutrients.

Eat Healthy. Be Healthy at Any Age.

When you have health challenges – which means you do not have an efficiently running body – they are likely due to toxic buildup in your body. Built-up plaque in the intestines can hinder nutrients from entering the bloodstream and being delivered where needed. Excess toxins build up in the liver and are deposited in the lymph nodes and fat cells. The fat cells can get fatter, and that's when you get fatter. The lymph nodes get clogged up and the toxins become trapped in the body. Then the liver needs detoxification. You can detoxify your liver and your body by doing an internal cleansing such as The Mini-Cleanse and The Cleansing Program provided in this book.

These are the Four Essential Steps to Good Health:

1. **Commitment to Health**. When your thoughts are focused on a specific outcome, you can accomplish what you want with ease. The Three Principles of Success will keep you focused on your goals (see Chapter 9).

2. **Internal Cleansing**. Cleansing the body removes toxins and is the foundation for good health. The Mini-Cleanse and The Cleansing Program in this book will get you started on your way to good health.

3. **Balanced Nutrition**. Adding proper nutrients through healthy foods and appropriate supplements continually repairs the body and keeps it healthy. The Maintenance Program in this book can help the body heal naturally without drugs.

4. **Regular Exercise**. Exercise is essential to keep muscles and bones strong, support good health, and energize the body. Exercise also removes toxic buildup in the lymphatic system through movement and sweating.

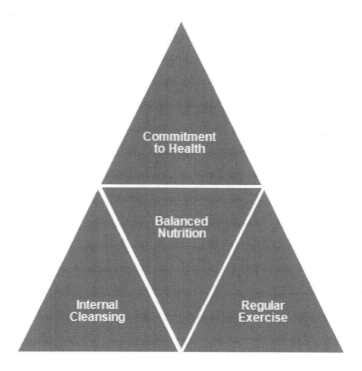

With knowledge comes power – the power to make healthy decisions about the food you eat. If you are experiencing health challenges, you may well be missing important nutrients. Proper food choices can help heal chronic health conditions.

Chapter 4
Carbohydrates: The Body's Fuel

Sustaining Health with Food Nutrients

Carbohydrates are in all plant foods: vegetables, leafy greens, fruits, grains, legumes, nuts, and seeds. They also occur in dairy products in the form of lactose, as well as in sweets like desserts, snacks, and sugar.

The two main types of carbohydrates are simple carbohydrates and complex carbohydrates. Simple carbohydrates are found in refined sugar – the white sugar used in cereals, desserts, fruit juices, and dairy products. The best foods from which to get simple carbohydrates are fruits because they contain fiber and important nutrients like vitamins and minerals.

Complex carbohydrates break down in the body more slowly. These are the starches that contain dietary fiber such as foods made from grains, like breads, pasta, and rice; legumes (beans and peas); and starchy vegetables like yams and squash.

If you have been diagnosed with insulin resistance, metabolic syndrome, or type II diabetes, read on!

Sustaining Health with Balanced Nutrition

Carbohydrates are also categorized as refined or unrefined. Refined carbohydrates such as white flour and white rice have had their fiber and nutrients removed. Unrefined carbohydrates such as whole grains, legumes, nuts, and seeds retain the vitamins, minerals, and fiber from the plants they come from.

Your body converts both refined and unrefined carbohydrates into simple sugars such as glucose that are absorbed by the bloodstream. The pancreas releases insulin, a hormone, to move glucose into your cells for energy. Medical science considers carbohydrates the body's chief source of energy, contributing four calories for every gram processed by the body.

An overabundance of carbohydrates causes too much sugar for the body to deal with, initiating a discharge of more insulin into your blood and tissues, which causes inflammation and disorders like insulin resistance, metabolic syndrome, and type II diabetes.

The standard American diet (SAD) includes about 50 percent to 60 percent carbohydrates, with more than half coming from refined, processed foods and sugars. These foods come in many forms: white flour, white rice, potatoes, breads, pizza, cereals, pancakes, waffles, ice cream, cookies, pastries, cakes, pies, sugar, candy, sodas, snacks, junk foods, and prepackaged meals. Refined carbohydrates are in many restaurant foods, also.

We develop cravings for refined carbohydrates, resulting in weight gain. These foods also lack many B vitamins and minerals needed for health, and can cause high blood pressure, heart disease, diabetes, obesity, and cancer.

Sylvia came to me fifty pounds overweight with cravings for sugar and processed foods. She and her

Eat Healthy. Be Healthy at Any Age.

family ate at fast-food restaurants several times
a week and they were all overweight. She had
low energy, felt fat and bloated, and began to see
signs of unhealthy physical conditions in her body.
Her doctor told her she had prediabetes and was
going to give her medication to relieve some of her
symptoms. That is when she came to me for help.

I assessed Sylvia's diet and analyzed her blood.
I showed her how the foods she ate contributed
to her being overweight, her health conditions,
and an imbalance in her blood. I taught her
the importance of balanced nutritional intake
through eating a wholesome diet instead of a diet
full of refined foods. That was when she decided
to make a commitment to her health and change
the way she was eating, living, and thinking
about food.

I offered Sylvia the Four Essential Steps to Good
Health above. It wasn't easy at first, but she
followed The Cleansing Program for two weeks,
and lost twelve pounds and fifteen inches around
the middle of her body. Sylvia now follows The
Maintenance Program, almost 100 percent, as a
lifetime eating plan. After five months, she has
lost forty-two pounds and has more energy for
daily tasks and family outings. Her blood values
have also improved. Her doctor was surprised to
see her weight loss and health changes.

Carbohydrates in the form of sugars added to foods and
drinks can cause sugar cravings and addiction. Even
fruits and starchy vegetables such as potatoes, beets,
and corn can cause you to crave additional sugary
foods and carbohydrates. We loosely call carbohydrates
"comfort foods" – *satisfying the addiction* is what
comforts us.

The major sources of added sugar in our food supply are sugar itself, regular soft drinks, candy, cakes, cookies, pies, fruit drinks, desserts, ice cream, sweetened yogurt, sweetened milk drinks, and grain products such as breads, pastas, cinnamon toast, cereals, and waffles.

The names for added sugars on food labels are agave nectar, beet sugar, brown sugar, cane sugar, confectionary sugar, corn sugar, corn sweetener, corn syrup, dehydrated cane juice, dextrin, dextrose (and many others ending in -*ose* such as fructose, lactose, and maltose), evaporated cane juice, fruit juice concentrate, high-fructose corn syrup (HFCS), honey, invert sugar, isomalt, malt syrup, maltodextrin, mannitol, maple syrup, molasses, raw sugar, rice syrup, sorbitol, sorghum, sugar, and xylitol.

Dr. Mary Enig, in her well-researched book, *Know Your Fats: The Complete Primer for Understanding the Nutrition of Fats, Oils and Cholesterol,* states that the more carbohydrates you eat, the more fat your liver and adipose tissue (connective tissue in which fat is stored) make. The result of excess carbohydrates is fat stored in the body.[1] This is true even if you stick to the healthier complex carbohydrates. Though they assimilate more slowly than simple carbohydrates, they still break down to sugar and are stored in fat cells if unused. When you deprive your body of sugar, there is no sugar to burn, and your body burns fat, another source of energy. If you want to lose weight, cutting down on starchy and sugary carbohydrates is the best first step, along with exercising to use up any excess sugar in your system.

Low-carbohydrate diets can change your body's metabolism and make it burn fat. But if you increase animal protein consumption while on a low-carbohydrate diet, there is a risk of kidney or liver trouble. Instead of

27

adding more animal protein, eat more green vegetables. They have more protein in the form of amino acids than starchy vegetables and are high in fiber.

Sugar is the favorite food of yeast in the body. When you eat products that break down into sugar or include sugar, you feed and encourage yeast growth in your body. Yeast is not what you want to see when you look at your live blood through a microscope; it contributes to a chain reaction to poor health and chronic conditions.

If you know you have candida (a type of yeast commonly found in the body), you should eliminate fruits, foods and drinks that contain added sugars, alcohol, dairy products, and all products that contain yeast (added yeast is found in processed and canned foods, breads, pizza, cheese, and desserts, to name just a few), and minimize starchy carbohydrate intake until your symptoms are gone. You want to deprive the body of the yeast's food. This may take one to two months.

Want to Lose Weight?

As mentioned above, when you want to lose weight, refined foods and starchy and sugary carbohydrates are what you want to remove from your diet until you reach your weight goal. Then you can slowly add low-sugar fruits, legumes, some grains, and low-starch vegetables such as yams and winter squash. If you start to gain weight and you are following a healthy eating plan, minimize grains until you find the right amount that will maintain your healthy weight. This is usually no more than 25 percent of each meal.

Keeping your blood sugar balanced preserves your energy and controls your weight. Type II diabetes, being overweight, lethargy, and obesity are some of the results of an imbalance. They are caused by eating carbohydrates such as sugar, sweet foods, dried fruit, refined flours such as in baked snacks and desserts, white bread, and white pasta. Foods with a low glycemic index (GI) help balance blood sugar.

Glycemic Index

The glycemic index rates a serving of food according to its effect on your body's blood sugar. Eating the wrong carbohydrates is the cause of many blood sugar imbalances. Low-fiber and processed foods raise blood sugar quickly. These foods have a high GI rating, between 100 and 150. By contrast, high-fiber foods and whole foods move slowly through the body, barely raise blood sugar at all, and allow for consistent blood sugar levels. These foods have a low GI rating, between 10 and 60. Using the glycemic index in choosing foods is another way to lessen health risks by controlling your weight and balancing your blood sugar levels. See the list of glycemic index foods and ratings in Appendix 1.

Calories

Calories are the amount of energy your body uses and produces from food. Carbohydrates provide four calories of energy for every gram you eat; fats provide nine calories per gram; and proteins provide four calories per gram. The USDA suggests that women eat around 2,000 calories per day and men around 2,500. You can easily increase these amounts by eating a high-fat diet, because fats contain over twice as many calories per gram as carbohydrates and proteins. Too much fat in your diet makes it difficult for your body to burn those calories. When this happens, the fat goes into the fat cells. That's how you become overweight.

Eat Healthy. Be Healthy at Any Age.

Fast foods, processed foods, and packaged foods are high in calories. They contain added sugars, fats, and salt to enhance their flavor. It's enlightening to read Nutrition Facts labels to determine the number of calories in one serving. Don't be deceived; Nutrition Facts labels are often based on a deceptive serving size! If the label shows 200 calories for a half-cup serving, and a natural serving is closer to one cup, you're getting a double whammy of calories in your serving. Restaurant food does not come with labels, so be very cautious about serving size when eating out.

How Much Carbohydrate Should You Eat?

There is no need to count carbohydrate grams or calories if you eat balanced meals consisting of whole foods high in fiber – vegetables; greens; some starchy vegetables, grains, legumes, nuts, and seeds – and low in sugar and fat. The more high-fiber foods you eat, the more full you will feel, and your calorie intake will be lower.

Chapter 5
Fats: The Real Truth

Another macronutrient is fat, an important part of our diet. In liquid form, fat is oil. In solid form, it is butter, grease, and shortening. Eating too much fat and the wrong fats make us fat. Eating good fats has many benefits:

- Fat gives the body its curves and is used for fuel when food intake is reduced.
- Fat prevents heat loss and protects us from temperature changes outside the body.
- Fat absorbs the fat-soluble vitamins – A, D, E, K – and carotenoids, a plant nutrient.
- Fat improves the flavor and texture of foods and provides a feeling of fullness.
- As an energy source, fat provides nine calories for every gram of fat consumed.

The building blocks of fat are fatty acids. Fatty acids look like linked chains under the microscope. They can be short, medium, or long chains depending on the number of links they contain. Just like a sponge full of water, fatty acids fill up with hydrogen. When a fatty acid is full, it is *saturated*. When not full, it is *unsaturated*. Hence the terms *saturated fats* and *unsaturated fats*. Saturated fats are long chains.

Coconut oil, which contains some saturated fat, is a medium chain. It is nutritionally different from pure saturated fat. Coconut oil is not harmful to the body like the saturated fats from animals and their by-products, unless it is refined.

Unsaturated Fats

Unsaturated fats in our food supply are polyunsaturated fats and monounsaturated fats. Polyunsaturated fats are liquid at room temperature and when refrigerated. There are two families of polyunsaturated fats: omega-6 and omega-3. Let's take a look at the "bad" fats and the "good" fats and how they affect our diet.

Bad Fats

Omega-6 Polyunsaturated Fats

Omega-6 fatty acids come from polyunsaturated oils extracted from seeds, such as sunflower, safflower, grape, pumpkin, and sesame; nuts, such as walnuts and butternuts; and vegetables, such as corn and soybeans. They provide linolenic acid (LA) which is abundant in processed foods and comes from refined oils. The harmful effects of these refined oils occur because they are highly unstable and become rancid in the body. When something turns rancid, it opens the door to free radical growth. To curb the effects of these oils, the food industry refines them, and it's the refining process that makes them bad for our health.

Free radicals are unstable molecules that react quickly with other compounds. They try to capture needed electrons from body cells to gain stability. A free radical attacks the nearest stable molecule, stealing its electron. When the attacked molecule loses its electron, it becomes a free radical itself, looking for an electron to steal and causing a chain reaction. Once this cycle begins, it can cascade, finally disrupting a living cell that eventually dies, weakening your body.

Refined oils are polyunsaturated vegetable oils conventionally produced and mechanically pressed and treated with chemical solvents. They are then heated at high temperatures and filtered many times to deodorize them and remove impurities. Preservatives are then added to protect them from becoming rancid. Yum! You get to eat this. When ingested, these oils are stored in fat cells with other toxins. Your cells get sick, your body gets fat, and disease can develop.

Since the introduction of refined polyunsaturated oils in our food supply, we suffer more from degenerative disease than ever before. Refined oils come to us as safflower, corn, canola, sunflower, and peanut oils. We use these oils, along with hydrogenated oils, in many meals we prepare at home. They are also in restaurant and convenience foods. Cleaning out your pantry and cupboards of these oils is a good idea.

Saturated Fats

Saturated fats are usually solid at room temperature. The main sources are animal products like red meat, poultry, and their by-products such as eggs, milk, yogurt, butter, cheese, and ice cream. Saturated fats also come from tropical plants and include coconut butter, coconut oil, palm kernel oil, and palm oil, but these have different properties than fats from animals, and are discussed later in this chapter.

You may have heard that saturated fats contribute to high cholesterol and heart disease. Cholesterol is built-up plaque in the arteries that minimizes normal blood flow. This can cause blockages that lead to heart attack and stroke. If you don't eat "manufactured" animals or their byproducts, you are eliminating the saturated fat and therefore the cholesterol that causes heart disease. Though your body needs a minimal amount of saturated fat, you can get it from the carbohydrates in plants rather than by eating animal products that contain high amounts. Cholesterol is naturally produced by your body and does not need to come from outside food sources.

Dr. Elton Haas, who wrote *Staying Healthy with Nutrition: The Complete Guide to Diet and Nutitional Medicine*, states that cholesterol in the blood results in oxidation and free radical damage. But total dietary fat is more problematic than cholesterol from food. The more bad fat you consume, the more potential health challenges you will face. It is important to increase exercise, fiber, and plant food intake. Plants contain antioxidants and phytonutrients that reduce inflammation and oxidation, increase good cholesterol, and protect the immune system.[1]

There is a solution to the saturated fat and cholesterol issue. Eat whole plant foods. Plants have no cholesterol and little saturated fat, if any.

Good Fats

An omega-6 fatty acid that is different from those found in the bad fats is found in oils that produce gamma-linolenic acid (GLA), which many health professionals consider beneficial. They include black current oil, which also contains omega-3 fatty acids; evening primrose oil; and borage seed oil. They are helpful for skin irritations and immune support. You will not find these oils in your food, nor will you cook with them. You can only buy them as supplements or in bottles in the refrigerated section of health food stores.

Omega-3 Polyunsaturated Fats

Omega-3 fatty acids are *essential* fatty acids, meaning the body cannot make them. We consume them in the food we eat. Omega-3 oils are beneficial oils. They provide anti-inflammatory support, nourish cells, and help regulate hormones and the nervous system. They protect us from heart disease, help with memory, and may help detoxify some cancers.

Omega-3 fatty acids come in many plant foods, supplying our body with alpha-linolenic acid (ALA), which is good for us. Omega-3 fatty acids are the healthiest of the fats and are the easiest to metabolize. They are found in the highest quantities in dark green leafy vegetables, broccoli, sea vegetables, and oils extracted from selected seeds such as flax, chia, and hemp seeds. Small amounts are also available in nuts and soybeans. Over 50 percent of the fat in flax seed oil and chia seed oil contains omega-3 fatty acids. But omega-3 oils are sensitive to heat, and become rancid, oxidize, and form free radicals when used in cooking or left unrefrigerated. It's best to get your omega-3 fatty acids from plants and whole seeds rather than from their oils because plants provide fiber as well, and fats are more effectively metabolized with fiber present.

The ALA from omega-3 fatty acids can be converted to eicosapentaenoic acid (EPA) in the body, but in many cases this is difficult to achieve. EPA and docosahexaenoic acid (DHA) are important in lowering the risk of coronary heart disease by lowering blood triglyceride and cholesterol levels, and they improve vision and brain activity. EPA and DHA can come directly from eating fish, fish oil, or microalgae. Although eating fish supplies omega-3 fatty acids, EPA, and DHA to the body, fish do not produce these fatty acids; they come from the foods that fish eat – plants and microalgae.

Here are the omegas in a nutshell:

Type of Fatty Acid	Name	Sources
Omega-6 fatty acids	linolenic acid (LA)	oils and seeds of sunflower, safflower, grape, pumpkin, and sesame; walnuts, butternuts, corn, soybeans
Omega-6 fatty acids	gamma-linolenic acid (GLA)	black currant oil, borage oil, evening primrose oil, breast milk
Omega-3 fatty acids	alpha-linolenic acid (ALA)	dark green leafy vegetables; broccoli; sea vegetables; flax, chia, and hemp oils; walnuts; soybeans
Omega-3 fatty acids	eicosapentaenoic acid (EPA) docosahexaenoic acid (DHA)	fatty fish – salmon, tuna, trout, herring, bluefish, sardines, mackerel; microalgae, fish oil

Monounsaturated Fat

Monounsaturated fats are usually liquid at room temperature and semi-solid when refrigerated. They provide protection against chronic diseases and are considered beneficial. They are found in olives, avocados, and most nuts, excluding walnuts and butternuts. Cold-pressed olive and avocado oils are great sources of monounsaturated fat, and they're minimally processed.

Coconut Oil

Remember that tropical oils (coconuts, coconut oil, coconut butter, palm oil, and palm kernel oil) are the only plant oils that contain saturated fats. Palm oil and palm kernel oil are heated at high temperatures and added to processed foods. We are told to stay away from tropical oils because they increase cholesterol levels, clog arteries, and eventually kill us with heart disease or stroke. But is this true for coconut oil?

Tropical populations consume large amounts of coconuts along with their natural oils. And studies done in the South Pacific islands show that heart disease is rare there, and do not confirm that coconuts and their oils have harmful effects on the population.[2]

Coconuts and their oils contain fatty acid chains of medium length, which are different from the long-chain saturated fats that cause damage to our arteries. Coconuts and their oils contain about 40 percent lauric acid. The body converts lauric acid into monolaurin, which acts as an antiviral, antimicrobial, and antifungal, destroying harmful microorganisms in the body. Coconuts can be a powerful tool in fighting immune diseases such as diabetes and rheumatoid arthritis.

The Worst Fats

Trans-fats

Trans-fats are plentiful in our food supply. Trans-fats are unsaturated oils put through a hydrogenation process in which hydrogen and vegetable oil spins at a rapid rate to form a solid fat. Nearly 90 percent of trans-fats in foods come from hydrogenated or partially hydrogenated oils. Hydrogenation makes food more stable, changes the texture, increases shelf life, and preserves freshness. Hydrogenated oils are widely used in the fast-food industry and in restaurants for deep-frying. The remaining 10 percent of trans-fats in our foods come from meat, dairy products, and a minute amount found naturally in some vegetables.

Eat Healthy. Be Healthy at Any Age.

Trans-fats are highly refined, heated, and filtered using chemicals. They can raise total cholesterol and lower HDL ("good") cholesterol. They are a manufactured, unnatural product harmful to the body, and cannot benefit health. Your body cannot metabolize trans-fats. They park themselves in the fat cells in your belly, hips, butt, and breasts, causing weight gain, obesity, and arterial disease.

The US Department of Agriculture shows that the trans-fats in our food supply come from:

Food	Percentage
Cakes, cookies, crackers, pies, bread, etc.	40%
Animal products	21%
Margarine	17%
Fried potatoes	8%
Potato chips, corn chips, popcorn	5%
Household shortening	4%
Breakfast cereal and candy	5%

Fred had a heart attack a few years before I met him. He was determined to change the course of his heart condition. His doctor tested his blood and wanted him to lower his cholesterol and triglyceride levels. Fred wanted to do it naturally without drugs. He started eating a plant-based diet, but still needed to make more changes to bring his blood values back to acceptable levels.

Fred came to me for a blood analysis. The analysis showed an imbalance due to dietary and nutritional deficiencies. I taught him about eating whole natural foods, and changing the kinds of fats and grains he was eating.

Fred made changes in his food choices and called me a few months later to tell me his doctor was happy with his new blood tests, and that an added benefit was that he now weighed what he had in high school. He thanked me for helping him with his goal.

Summary of Good Oils and Fats

Good fats are:

- Black current oil, evening primrose oil, and borage seed oil
- Omega-3 fatty acids from dark green leafy vegetables; broccoli; sea vegetables; flax, chia, and hemp seeds; walnuts; and soybeans
- Extra virgin olive oil, which is best added to foods after cooking, drizzled on soups and vegetables in place of butter, or used in salad dressings
- Avocado and coconut oils, which tolerate higher cooking temperatures. Use them for sautéing your foods and on vegetables before you roast them in the oven.

Chapter 6
Protein: The Treasured Nutrient

Protein is essential for good health. It is a primary component of our muscles, hair, nails, skin, eyes, and internal organs. We need to consume protein regularly for growth and maintenance of body tissues. Most people think animal products make up the protein in our diet. The cattle industry, dairy industry, poultry industry, and government food groups condition us to believe this through their advertising. But is it true?

A Case for Plant Protein

Protein from animal sources does not make protein in your body; the amino acids in your body make the protein that the body uses. Amino acids come from plant foods and the plants in animals' diets that you ingest by eating animals. The protein in animals and their by-products must convert to amino acids before your body can use it efficiently. This conversion takes time and energy, making it an inefficient way to provide your body with protein. When protein comes to you through plant foods, it is readily available in the form of amino acids.

Your body needs at least twenty-two known amino acids to keep it healthy. Living cells in the body use amino acids to build muscle, repair cells and tissues, and preserve the health of the body. At least eight amino acids that are essential to your health must come from plants, animals that eat plants, or animals that eat other plant-eating animals.

Many plant proteins contain beneficial levels of these essential amino acids while being low in one or two. This is why intake of various kinds of plants is important in ensuring you are getting all the essential amino acids. The most plentiful protein in plant foods comes from beans, grains, leafy greens, vegetables, nuts, seeds, olives, sea vegetables, avocados, and green super food powders.

Dairy Products and Osteoporosis

When sufficient quantities of precious alkaline minerals are not available from food, your body takes them from bones, teeth, and tissues, contributing to osteoporosis, arthritis, heart disease, stroke, and cancer.

Osteoporosis is a disease of the bones. It occurs mostly in women who are postmenopausal, but it affects men as well. When estrogen levels decline as we get older, the risk of developing this disease can increase. Many believe osteoporosis points to a calcium shortage. Our doctors tell us to take calcium supplements and eat dairy products to curb the loss of calcium and prevent osteoporosis.

The dairy industry encourages consumption of their products to increase calcium and build strong bones. But is this working? A study of American women aged fifty and older shows a high rate of hip fractures and the worst bone health in the world.[1] The protein and phosphorous (an acid mineral) content in dairy products can cancel the beneficial effects of calcium and ultimately *contribute* to osteoporosis.

The body does not produce calcium on its own. It must come from outside sources through the food we eat or through supplements. But the body will not absorb calcium unless many other vitamins and minerals are present to aid absorption. If you are not getting a balance of nutrients, you are not getting enough calcium, either.

> Mary was diagnosed with osteopenia, a condition that is usually a precursor to osteoporosis. After many years of taking medication to stave off its progression, Mary was diagnosed with osteoporosis. She stopped taking the medication. She participated in weight training to build stronger bones, but she was concerned about her diet and what supplements to take in order to improve the condition.
>
> Mary was in her late fifties when she came to me for a dietary assessment. She ate a high-protein diet with low vegetable intake, which can cause a decrease of alkaline minerals from the body. After six months of weight training and eating foods that provide more minerals, Mary's condition improved.

In *Traditional Foods Are Your Best Medicine: Improving Health and Longevity with Native Nutrition,* Dr. Ronald Schmid writes about studies done by Dr. Weston Price on several groups who ate dairy products. One group – the people of the Loetschental Valley – drank raw, whole milk and ate both fresh and cultured cheese and butter. They lived long and healthy lives without chronic disease. The milk was not pasteurized or homogenized, and it came from healthy, grass-fed, well-exercised animals.

The quality of their food was clearly responsible for the presence of a rich number of nutrients.[2]

Today we pasteurize and homogenize dairy products. Pasteurization changes the chemical structures of proteins and fats in milk and destroys harmful bacteria at the expense of healthful enzymes lost during the heating process. Homogenization is a blending process that keeps milk and cream from separating. Synthetic vitamin D is added, resulting in another manufactured, processed product that is challenging to your health.

Cheese, ice cream, and butter are highly condensed products from milk.

- 1 ounce of cheese is equivalent to 8 to 10 ounces of milk
- 1 pound of hard cheese is equivalent to about 5 quarts of milk
- 1 gallon of ice cream is equivalent to about 5.5 quarts of milk
- 1 pound of butter is equivalent to about 9.6 quarts of milk

Manufactured cows ingest insecticides, drugs, hormones, antibiotics, and pesticides in their food supply. These substances show up in their milk and become part of your body when you consume dairy products. Grass-fed, chemical-free animals do not pass these additives to you. Are poor-quality man-made foods causing chronic diseases that are widespread in our society today? The answer is likely *yes*!

Toxic Chemicals in Animal Protein

Pan-frying, broiling, and barbequing use high heat to cook meat. These methods produce high levels of heterocyclic amines (HCA) and polycyclic aromatic

Eat Healthy. Be Healthy at Any Age.

hydrocarbons (PAC), which form the carcinogenic compounds that produce cancer-causing tumors. Eating foods cooked this way, or their juices, can cause colon cancer. Beware if you like to grill your meats.

The best cooking methods are boiling, steaming, stewing, poaching, and braising, at temperatures under 212 degrees and without browning beforehand. Plant foods do not produce HCAs or PACs unless they are burned.

Nitrates and nitrites are added to processed foods to preserve them and provide a reddish color. They are added to sausage, hot dogs, bacon, and cold cuts, which would be grey in color without these carcinogenic chemicals. These chemicals are also added to livestock feed, cheese products (those preserved with pickling salt), nonfat dry milk, some fish, fish by-products, and beer. When cooked at high temperatures, these foods produce nitrosamines, another carcinogenic chemical.

The Hunter-Gatherer Diet or the Ancestral Diet

There is much buzz these days about the hunter-gatherer diet. One hundred years ago we did not have many of the diseases that are prevalent today. Foods in the days of the hunter-gatherer came from natural sources – the land and healthy grazing animals. Today's diet consists mostly of manufactured animals and packaged and processed foods. Although the food industry has made preparing meals more convenient, foods of the past were certainly healthier.

How Much Protein Does a Body Need?

Your body is about 7 percent protein. It doesn't need more than 7 percent protein from food to sustain good health. In fact, Dr. T. Colin Campbell, in his book *The China Study: Startling Implications for Diet, Weight Loss and Long-Term Health,* specifically links chronic diseases to the consumption of animal protein. His research proves that a plant-based diet improves health and can often reverse disease.[3] Dr. Campbell suggests we only need 3 percent to 5 percent protein in our daily diet. Plant foods can easily provide this amount if you eat enough food and a variety of plants each day.

The Recommended Dietary Allowance (RDA) of protein for both men and women is 0.8 grams per kilogram of body weight.[4] Here is how to calculate your RDA for protein in grams:

> Body weight in pounds divided by 2.2 = weight in kilograms × 0.8.

Examples:

130 lbs. ÷ 2.2 = 59 kilograms
× 0.8 = 47.27 grams of protein per day

150 lbs. ÷ 2.2 = 68 kilograms
× 0.8 = 54.54 grams of protein per day

175 lbs. ÷ 2.2 = 79.5 kilograms
× 0.8 = 63.63 grams of protein per day

To put this in perspective, here is a list of grams of protein from cooked animal products:

Protein from Cooked Animal Products

Food	Quantity	Protein (grams)
Beef, top sirloin	3 oz.	23
Chicken breast w/skin	½ breast	29
Chicken thigh w/skin	1 thigh	16

Eat Healthy. Be Healthy at Any Age.

Food	Quantity	Protein (grams)
Crab, Alaskan king	1 leg	26
Egg, white and yolk	2	13
Milk, whole	1 cup	8
Salmon or trout, cooked	4 oz.	14
Tuna, fresh cooked	3 oz.	12
Turkey breast w/skin	3 ½ oz.	29

As you can see, three ounces of beef (a small serving) is half the daily requirement for a 130-pound person. A steak ordered at a restaurant is usually four to five ounces for a small serving and up to eight ounces for a standard serving. Americans consume one-and-a-half to four times more animal protein than they need each day. And research has shown that the RDA is about 50 percent more protein than the body needs for good health!

Here is a sample menu that shows how much protein and calcium you can consume in one day eating plant-based foods:

Sample Menu for One Day

	Quantity	Protein (grams)	Calcium (mgs.)
Breakfast			
Grapefruit	½	.95	27
Oatmeal	1 cup	5.7	125
Almond milk	½ cup	.5	0
Sliced almonds	1 oz.	6.2	61
Lunch			
Butter lettuce salad	3 cups	2.22	57.6
Tomatoes	1 cup	1.6	18
Avocado	½	2	12

Cucumber	½	1	24
White beans	½ cup	7.5	23
Olive oil/lemon juice	0	0	
Snack			
Almond butter	2 Tbsp.	4.8	86.4
Celery sticks	2 large	1.4	80
Dinner			
Mixed vegetables	3 cups	6	120
Brown and Wild Rice	1 cup	4.5	11.7
Olive oil and herbs	0	0	
Salad	dinner size	3	60
Totals		**47.37 grams**	**705.7 milligrams**

As you can see, there is enough protein in this plant-based meal plan for a 130-pound person. You would not be likely to develop a protein deficiency eating plant foods. You would ingest usable protein in the form of amino acids, with plenty of absorbable calcium from natural sources, and not gain weight.

Take a look at the chart below to see how much protein and calcium is available from plant-based foods.

Protein and Calcium Found in Selected Plant Foods

Food	Quantity	Protein (grams)	Calcium (milligrams)
Asparagus	1 cup	4.3	41
Almonds	1 oz.	6.2	61
Almond butter	1 tbsp.	2.4	43.2
Avocado	1 med.	4	24
Beans			
Black	1 cup	15	46
Lentils	1 cup	17.2	38

Eat Healthy. Be Healthy at Any Age.

Food	Quantity	Protein (grams)	Calcium (milligrams)
Navy	1 cup	17	150
Broccoli, florets	1 cup	2.9	45
Cauliflower	1 cup	2.2	31
Cucumber, medium	1	2	48
Green beans	1 cup	2.4	59
Greens			
Bok choy, cooked	1 cup	2.3	141
Collard greens, cooked	1 cup	2.7	181
Kale, raw	1 cup	2.2	90
Spinach, cooked	1 cup	5.3	244
Grains			
Brown and wild rice	1 cup	4.5	11.7
Buckwheat noodles	½ cup	8	
Millet, cooked	1 cup	6.5	5.2
Quinoa, cooked	1 cup	8.1	31.5
Spelt pasta, whole grain	1 cup	8	
Brown rice pasta	1 cup	4	
Whole wheat bread	1 reg. slice	2.5	25.7
Whole wheat pasta	1 cup	7.4	21
Seeds			
Chia	1 oz.	4.4	179
Hemp	3 tbsp.	11	
Pumpkin	1 oz.	7	12
Sunflower	1 oz.	5.9	22
Sesame	1 tbsp.	1.6	88
Tofu, firm, Vitasoy	2.79 oz.	7.031	98.8

Some people tell me they require animal protein in their diet. They feel better, can overcome hunger pangs, and sustain their energy level longer. They say animal protein works for them, and I understand this sentiment. I ate animal protein and low carbohydrates for some time. It sustained me for several hours during the day. But I had issues with bad breath, body odor, and constipation during this time. When I changed what I ate to high-fiber foods, those issues were eliminated. The added fiber made me feel full and sustained me for many hours. Eating too much animal protein can cause chronic and debilitating diseases. It is time to look at animal foods and plant foods differently.

According to a study published in the former *Journal of the American Dietetic Association*, vegetarians were slimmer; had higher intakes of fiber, vitamins, and minerals; and consumed less saturated fat and cholesterol. The study concluded that vegetarian diets are associated with lower risks of disease.[5] Protein deficiencies are not associated with plant-based diets, and diseases of excess are associated with too much animal protein. Fresh, plant-based foods are the healthiest sources of protein for your body.

Chapter 7
Micronutrients: The Workhorses of Health

Vitamins, minerals, antioxidants, and phytonutrients are micronutrients. They come from the carbohydrates, fats, and proteins in the foods we eat. They are essential to good health.

Vitamins

Vitamins are essential compounds needed in small amounts for body function and health. Each vitamin performs a certain purpose. They aid macronutrients by converting food into energy and body tissue. Too much of any one vitamin can be toxic. Too little of any one vitamin can cause a deficiency in the body. A balanced diet including a variety of foods supplies the vitamins needed for building and repairing every cell in the body, and for keeping the body consistently healthy.

There are two types of vitamins: water-soluble and fat-soluble. Water-soluble vitamins are vitamin C and the B vitamin group. They dissolve in water, absorb water, and mix with our blood. They are easily eliminated through urine when not needed. Fat-soluble vitamins – A, D, E, and K – need fat for absorption. They are stored in the liver for later use.

Vitamins vital to good health are vitamins A, C, D, E, K, and the B vitamins. The list below provides their chemical names, functions, and many of their sources.

Fat-Soluble Vitamin	Functions	Sources
A and beta-carotene (an antioxidant)	Support healthy skin, eyes, bones teeth, hair, immune function.	Beta-carotene converts these foods into vitamin A: green, yellow, and orange vegetables such as carrots, cantaloupe, apricots, sweet potatoes, squashes, green leafy vegetables, spinach, broccoli
D_3 (cholecalciferol) D_2 (synthetic form)	Aid absorption of calcium and phosphorus. Needed for strong bones, muscles, teeth, healthy skin.	Sunlight on skin, salmon, herring, mackerel, eggs, supplements from animal hides
E (d-alpha tocopherol) (an antioxidant)	Helps protect cell membranes, lipoproteins, and fats from oxidation, supports immune function, helps form and protect red blood cells.	Almonds, almond milk, sunflower seeds, asparagus, leafy green vegetables, olive oil, olives, spinach
K	Needed for proper blood clotting and calcium regulation.	Green vegetables, dark leafy greens

Eat Healthy. Be Healthy at Any Age.

Water-Soluble Vitamin	Functions	Sources
C (ascorbic acid) (an antioxidant)	Supports bones, teeth, red blood cell formation, healing wounds and cuts; fights infection; aids absorption of iron.	Oranges, grapefruit, lemons, strawberries, raspberries, cantaloupe, sweet peppers, broccoli, Brussels sprouts, tomatoes, green vegetables
B-1 (thiamine)	Needed for carbohydrate metabolism, muscle coordination, nervous system; boosts memory.	Fortified breakfast cereals, whole grains, wheat germ, legumes, nuts
B-2 (riboflavin)	Necessary for healthy skin and eyes; metabolizes protein, fat, carbohydrates; brings energy to cells; activates B3 and B6.	Whole grains, fortified breads and cereals, green vegetables, yams, legumes, almonds, pumpkin seeds
B-3 (niacin)	Aids in maintenance of skin, nervous system, mental functioning; metabolizes food for energy; releases stored calcium.	Whole grains, cereal, legumes, nuts, avocado
B-5 (pantothenic acid)	Needed for normal functioning of adrenal glands, helps free energy from carbohydrates and fats.	All plant foods.

Sustaining Health with Balanced Nutrition

Water-Soluble Vitamin	Functions	Sources
B-6 (pyridoxine)	Helps protein and fat metabolism and functioning of red blood cells and nervous system.	Fortified cereals, whole grains, legumes, seeds, green leafy vegetables, avocados, tomatoes. squashes, peas, split peas.
B-12 (cobalamin)	Needed for healthy nervous system, brain, energy, formation of red blood cells; builds genetic material.	Originates from bacteria. Animal products, fortified foods, supplements
Biotin	Helps metabolize amino acids, needed for normal hair and growth.	Legumes, whole grains, nut, seeds, vegetables
Choline	Used for memory and nerve and muscle function.	Flax seeds, sesame seeds, lentils, fish, leafy greens, cauliflower, potatoes, oats, wheat germ, supplemental lecithin
Folic Acid (folate)	Necessary for proper red blood cell formation, metabolism of fats, amino acids, genetic material.	Leafy greens, avocado, broccoli, legumes, seeds, whole grains, and many fruits and vegetables
Inositol	Needed for healthy cells in brain, bone marrow, eyes, hair, skin; lowers cholesterol.	Whole grains, wheat germ, lima beans, cabbage, cantaloupe, grapefruit, some nuts
PABA (para-aminobenzoic acid)	Important for skin, hair, intestines, red blood cells; used in sunscreen products.	Found naturally in most foods, whole grains, wheat germ

Minerals

Minerals are elements that come from the soil. We obtain most of our minerals from fruits, vegetables, and animals that eat plants. Minerals work together with vitamins, carbohydrates, proteins, and fats. Too much of one mineral can compete with absorption of another mineral. Too few minerals can cause a deficiency in the body.

Minerals are the basic building blocks of body material. They move through the blood into our cells for use by the body. There are well over one hundred known minerals. *Essential minerals* cannot be produced by your body in sufficient amounts to preserve good health, so you must obtain them from food. Here is a list of minerals, their functions, and food sources.

Mineral	Functions	Food Sources
Boron	Reduces calcium loss; bone health.	Leafy greens, nuts, legumes, avocados
Calcium	Builds bones and teeth; needed for muscles, nerves, heart function, alkaline balance.	Legumes, leafy greens such as kale, Chinese cabbage, green vegetables, almond, chia seeds, sesame seeds, tofu
Chloride	Maintains electrolyte balance in bodily fluids.	Sea salt, sea vegetables, celery, tomatoes, vegetables
Chromium	Regulates blood sugar, heart muscle, metabolism; storage of carbohydrates, fats, proteins.	Whole grains, fortified cereals, broccoli, some fruits and herbs
Cobalt	Red blood cell production; part of B^{12}	Leafy green vegetables, legumes, sea vegetables, fish

Sustaining Health with Balanced Nutrition

Mineral	Functions	Food Sources
Copper	Needed for protein metabolism, building hormones, blood production.	Nuts, seeds, legumes, tofu, raisons, whole grains
Fluoride	Healthy teeth and bones.	Seafood, tea, sea vegetables
Iodine	Normal thyroid function.	Sea vegetables – particularly kelp, ocean fish
Iron	Transports oxygen to tissues, production of energy, makes hemoglobin, helps with immune system.	Whole grains, seafood, legumes, leafy greens, fortified cereals
Magnesium	Healthy muscles, bones, teeth, nerves; energy production; alkaline balance.	Whole grains, leafy greens, green vegetables, legumes, nuts, seeds, lentils
Manganese	Healthy bones, metabolism of protein and carbohydrates.	Vegetables, tea, fortified cereals
Molybdenum	Processes proteins and other substances.	Whole grains, nuts, legumes
Phosphorus	Builds bones and teeth; needed for energy production, calcium absorption.	Most fruits, vegetables, cereals
Potassium	Regulates fluid balance and muscle contraction; alkaline balance.	Leafy green vegetables, avocados, green beans, broccoli, peas, tomatoes, potatoes, whole grains, nuts, seeds, salmon
Selenium	An antioxidant;, protects from free radical damage to all body cells.	Whole grains, Brazil nuts, seafood, seeds

Eat Healthy. Be Healthy at Any Age.

Mineral	Functions	Food Sources
Silicon	Helps form bone, cartilage, collagen, nails.	Found in plant fiber, avocado, cucumbers, onions, alfalfa, dark leafy greens
Sodium	Regulates fluid balance outside cells, nerve impulses, muscles; alkaline balance.	Processed foods, table salt. Healthier options: found naturally in most foods and sea salt
Sulfur	Builds hair, skin, nails.	Broccoli, cabbage, Brussels sprouts, kale, collard greens, onions, garlic, sea vegetables, nuts, raspberries
Vanadium	Sugar regulation in diabetics, improves body structure and lean body mass.	Olive oil, polyunsaturated vegetable oils, green beans, cabbage, carrots, oats, rice, buckwheat, dill, parsley
Zinc	Component of enzymes; wound healing, sexual function, insulin storage, carbohydrate metabolism.	Nuts and seeds, whole grains, beans, ginger root

Minerals are lost through cooking foods, and the body loses minerals from exercising, sweating, illness, laxatives, and surgery. It is important to eat mineral-rich foods daily. The mineral content of the soil in which plant foods are grown is important. When soil minerals are depleted, plants cannot absorb them. Sustainably farmed foods grown in mineral-rich soil contain sufficient minerals for good health. Most organic farms nourish their soil regularly. Eating a variety of mineral-rich plants balances mineral intake.

Antioxidants Help Defend against Disease

Antioxidants reduce the harmful effects of free radical damage. Free radicals have an unpaired number of electrons, making them unpredictable. They move through the body searching for an electron to steal from another cell to become stable. Cell damage occurs when free radicals merge with DNA or cell membranes. They make cells perform improperly and can cause cell death. Your body can become overpowered by free radicals, causing illness and disease. Antioxidants defend the body by turning off these unstable molecules before they can damage cells.

An example of free-radical corrosion is a cut apple, pear, avocado, or banana that turns brown from exposure to air (oxygen). Similar rusting can occur in your body. It is known by the medical community as *oxidative stress.* Free radicals can cause oxidative stress, which causes cell mutation, which causes cancer. Avoid free radical invaders by eating a lot of variously colored vegetables.

Toxins cause oxidation and free-radical damage in your body. Toxins exist in our air, water, homes, and gardens from pesticides, bacteria, fungus, mold, cigarette smoke, and alcohol, and are by-products of normal metabolism. When your body produces energy, it creates free radicals by using oxygen to break down the nutrients in food. Your body has ways of dealing with free-radical damage; it produces antioxidants from the foods you eat. Antioxidants supply electrons to free radicals to help ward off cellular change and prevent disease. Dietary antioxidants come from specific vitamins – A, C, E, and K. If you eat enough antioxidant-rich foods, these vitamins can combat the free-radical damage produced by them. Kale is an excellent example of an antioxidant-dense food that fights free-radical damage.

Eat Healthy. Be Healthy at Any Age.

More Antioxidants to Keep You Healthy

Other antioxidants are glutathione, lipoic acid, coenzyme Q-10, and selenium. When combined with vitamins C and E, they work synergistically to bring about greater free-radical mitigation. Each antioxidant has its own job to do in regard to protecting cells that cannot be done by other antioxidants.

Glutathione is important in neutralizing toxins in the liver from over-the-counter and prescribed drugs, chemicals added to processed foods such as luncheon meats and bacon, excessive alcohol use, and tobacco smoking. Glutathione also boosts the immune system. Glutathione levels decrease in your body as you age, but you can increase them by eating foods that contain glutathione – fruits and vegetables.

Lipoic acid helps control symptoms of stroke, heart disease, cataracts, diabetes, memory loss, aging, and cancer. Dr. L. Packer, who wrote *The Antioxidant Miracle: Put Lipoic Acid, Pycnogenol, and Vitamins E and C to Work for You,* maintains that it is the only antioxidant that can "recycle itself from free radical form back to its antioxidant form," giving it great benefit over other antioxidants.[1] Potatoes and spinach provide lipoic acid, and you can take supplements that provide it as well.

Vitamin E, another antioxidant, helps protect fats in cells from damage from oxidation that contributes to chronic degenerative diseases and aging. It helps prevent wrinkles and brown spots on your skin, and cancer. Vitamin E helps relieve symptoms of inflammatory conditions like arthritis, prevents cataracts, and reduces the risk of prostate and breast cancers. Vitamin E is present in fish oils and seafood such as haddock and herring. It is present in whole

58

grains that contain the bran where fiber and many other nutrients reside. Vitamin E is also found in nuts, seeds, and unrefined vegetable oils. Tocotrienol is the form of vitamin E found in bran cereals.

Vitamin C can prevent free-radical damage by protecting DNA, strengthening the immune system, and keeping viral infections at bay. It acts with vitamin E to prevent the damage that leads to heart disease. It is important in collagen production and keeping your skin from aging, and can help protect us from cataracts. Vitamin C is present in many fruits and vegetables, especially green and red ones. One of the best sources is citrus fruits – oranges, grapefruits, and lemons.

Selenium is a trace mineral found in soil. It works together with vitamin E to protect us from cancer, heart disease, and stroke. Selenium is found in various other foods – fish, shellfish, nuts, brown rice, and vegetables – and particularly in foods grown in selenium-treated soil.

Your body makes coenzyme Q-10. It is also found in oily fish such as salmon. Coenzyme Q-10 is necessary in producing energy. The process of producing energy creates free radicals and, as an antioxidant, coenzyme Q-10 reduces free radicals. It restores brain cells and maintains a healthy heart. Cholesterol-lowering drugs inhibit the manufacture of coenzyme Q-10 in the body; therefore, taking coenzyme Q-10 supplements can be helpful if you take statin drugs.

Phytonutrients Enhance Antioxidant Strength

Nature's pharmacy includes phytonutrients, or phytochemicals. These nutrients, found in plants, can boost the immune system, act as antioxidants, and help the body preserve healthy hormone levels. They occur in most fruits and vegetables. Eating a balance of fruits and vegetables can strengthen antioxidant defenses. Whole, natural foods are abundant in phytonutrients. A sampling of foods high in phytonutrients includes apples, berries, carrots, citrus fruits, cruciferous vegetables (cruciferous means "cross-bearing"; the flowers of these vegetables have four petals resembling a cross, such as cauliflower, cress, cabbage, bok choy, and broccoli), dried fruits, garlic, onions, greens, red grapes, wine, sesame oil, sesame seeds, soy foods, spinach, sweet potatoes, tomatoes, turmeric, walnuts, and winter squashes.

Flavonoids are compounds that occur naturally in the pigments of plants. They offset damage to the body from free radicals, boost the immune system, reduce inflammation in the body, defend against plaque buildup in the arteries, stabilize blood pressure, and can increase sexual performance in men. There are thousands of different flavonoids in plant foods. Here are some examples:

- Carotenoids come from yellow and orange plants like carrots and winter squashes.
- Chlorophyll comes from green plants like spinach, lettuces, green beans, and broccoli.
- Curcumin comes from yellow plants like corn, yellow peppers, and turmeric.
- Lycopene comes from red plants like tomatoes and watermelon.
- Bioflavonoids come from citrus fruits.

There are many phytonutrients, and it's not necessary to know the names of all of them. By varying your plant food choices each day, you can ingest the nutrients necessary to fight disease naturally.

Suzanne came to me after having a repeat bout of bronchitis. It seemed that several times a year she would get a horrible, hacking cough, resulting in a sore, burning, heavy chest. She normally took antibiotics for it, but they didn't seem to be working this time, so she came to me for help.

The best way to avoid chronic bronchitis is to eat an abundance of vegetables that provide antioxidants and phytonutrients. This helps the immune system control bacteria and virus growth. Suzanne's diet did not include many vegetables, so she added vegetables and eliminated animal protein.

I suggested she breathe a nebulizer containing a combination of liquid antioxidants three times a day, and her lungs felt better after using it the first time. I also recommended that she drink freshly made vegetable juices. Within a few days, she no longer needed the nebulizer.

Chapter 8
Non-Nutrients: The Essential Benefits

Fiber – Its Health-Giving Benefits

Fiber is the indigestible part of plant food. It moves through the body without adding calories or fat, offering many benefits to you. The higher the fiber content in a plant food, the better it is for you. Here are the benefits and roles fiber plays in your diet:

- Prevents constipation by increasing the volume of stool
- Helps remove wastes from your body
- Lowers cholesterol
- Balances blood sugar and insulin levels
- Controls the growth of bacteria in the colon lining
- Satisfies the appetite by making the stomach feel full

Fiber comes in two forms: insoluble and soluble. Insoluble fiber is known as cellulose and lignin. It does not dissolve in liquid. It moves bulk through the intestines and encourages regular bowel movements,

Sustaining Health with Balanced Nutrition

passing through the body quickly. You can find insoluble fiber in plant foods such as whole grains, vegetables, nuts, and seeds.

Soluble fiber absorbs liquids and moves slowly through the digestive tract. It causes you to feel full longer and helps balance your blood sugar level. Soluble fiber can help lower total cholesterol and LDL ("bad") cholesterol. It regulates blood sugar in diabetics and balances digestive problems in people with irritable bowel syndrome (IBS). You can find soluble fiber in plant foods such as oats, oat bran, barley, flax seeds, dried beans and peas, nuts, fruits, and cooked high-fiber vegetables such as yams, carrots, and dark leafy greens.

Many plant foods provide both insoluble and soluble fiber, so which fiber-rich vegetables you eat is not as important as eating enough total fiber for good health. The US Food and Drug Administration (FDA) recommends eating about 25 grams of fiber each day. But high cholesterol is still a major concern in the US, and laxatives are one of the biggest-selling over-the-counter medications, so I suggest getting more than 25 grams per day. Because insoluble fiber can cause bloating and gas, slowly build up to eating more insoluble fiber over a period of a few months.

Animal products do not supply fiber. Americans are accustomed to animal products being the largest portion of their meal, so is it any wonder that we lack fiber and suffer from constipation and colorectal cancer?

We talked about the glycemic index (GI) in the chapter about carbohydrates. This index is used to rate foods according to their effect on blood sugar. Low-fiber foods raise blood sugar quickly. High-fiber foods move slowly through your system, rarely raise blood sugar, and offer a better connection to good health. However, some conditions are triggered by too much fiber.

Eat Healthy. Be Healthy at Any Age.

Sara came to me after having painful digestive problems when she ate or drank certain foods. She knew certain foods triggered the pain, but after she was diagnosed with irritable bowel syndrome (IBS) she was confused about what dietary changes she should make to prevent this ongoing discomfort. She came to see me for help.

IBS is triggered by many kinds of foods, drinks, and chemical additives, particularly insoluble fiber foods such as beans, whole grains, cereals, and some vegetables. Insoluble fiber doesn't cause IBS, but it irritates the digestive system causing painful cramps, bloating, gas, and diarrhea. The soluble fiber that is available in foods such as rice, pasta, and sweet potatoes is a better choice with this condition. I suggested The Cleansing Program for a week to clean out her digestive system and start the healing process in the small intestines. After the week, Sara was without pain and relieved of the stress around food choices.

I taught Sara about IBS and outlined a maintenance dietary program to manage the healing process. She now eats in a balanced way that prevents discomfort, bloating, and diarrhea, and she has no more discomfort.

Here are some tips about fiber:

- *Increase fiber intake.* Fiber prevents cells from damage and helps absorb toxins, flushing them from the body. High-quality, high-fiber foods include vegetables, grains, beans, greens, fruits, nuts, and seeds. Adding more of these foods to your meals increases your fiber intake.
- *Eat whole foods and some whole grains.* Whole grains contain fiber, but they increase insulin production and can cause weight gain and

allergic reactions. Beans, for instance, are a better alternative than grains because they are protein-rich.

- *Reduce and eventually remove refined foods from your diet.* Refined foods come in many forms: white flour, white rice, breads, cereals, pancakes, waffles, ice cream, pastries, sugar, candy, cookies, sodas, snack and junk foods, and processed, prepackaged meals that are canned, boxed, or frozen. Refined foods contain chemical additives with low to no nutrient value or fiber, and are devoid of vitamins and minerals. They are poor dietary choices, leading to increased cholesterol levels and a high risk of developing heart disease.

By eating a variety of plant-based foods at every meal, you can get the fiber your system needs. Adding more fiber to your diet can help maintain your weight and reduce your risks for the top three diseases in our country today: heart disease, cancer, and stroke.

Water – The Key to Elimination of Toxins

Water is essential for life. It is important to your body's mineral and electrolyte balance. Electrolytes are mineral ions that produce and transfer electrical energy in the body, and they metabolize vitamins and enzymes. Water aids nutrients, oxygen, and other chemicals in moving to where they are needed in the body.

Your body consists of 70 percent or more water. Plasma and lymph fluids are over 90 percent water. Your body constantly loses water through urination, defecation, respiration, and perspiration, and you must replace the water in your body every day or your cells will dehydrate and die. Dehydration causes your body to age and your skin to wrinkle, and can threaten your life.

Toxins enter your body from our polluted environment. Drugs, beer, wine, and liquor act as poisons in your body. The FDA does not regulate these drinks or require them to carry ingredients labels. There are many toxic ingredients in these drinks such as ammonia, asbestos, and pesticide residues, to name a few. Water helps remove such toxins through the skin, lungs, kidneys, and colon.

Coffee and tea are diuretics and contain toxic substances. Diuretics increase the flow of urine, pulling water out of the body and causing dehydration and cell death.

Drinking clean water and eating fresh, raw fruits and vegetables supplies your body with what it needs for hydration. Cooking removes much of the water content in food. By eating more raw foods such as salads, fruits, and vegetables, you add water to your body in addition to healthy nutrients.

How much water should you drink?

To supply the body with enough water, you must drink about one quart of water for every fifty pounds of weight. If you weigh 150 pounds, you should drink three quarts of water every day. This is more water than the popular recommendations of eight cups a day or half an ounce for every pound of weight. Work up to one quart for every fifty pounds and you will notice a big difference in your energy level.

What kind of water should you drink?

You need to drink clean, pure water. Many of the bottled waters in stores today come from public water supplies, perhaps with the flavor enhanced to be more appealing.

The best water to drink is alkaline water. Alkaline water is available in bottles from local markets, but can be expensive. You can drink purified water, water filtered using reverse osmosis, filtered water with alkaline drops added, or ionized water.

You can buy an ionizer, which not only provides alkaline water, but water that acts as an antioxidant, challenging and eliminating free-radical growth. Ionized water provides a pH of 9.5 or better, and an oxidation reduction potential (ORP) of at least -250 millivolts. ORP measures the amount of millivolts of electrons in oxygen. The ORP reading can either be plus (+) or minus (-). A positive ORP reading shows the oxidizing properties of oxygen in water. A negative ORP reading shows antioxidant capacities in the water. Ionized water acts as an antioxidant that neutralizes free radicals. Look at my website, www.janefalke.com/antioxidants, for more information on the benefits of antioxidants.

Oxygen – It's Not All in the Air You Breathe

In 1931, Dr. Otto Warburg was awarded the Nobel Peace Prize. He discovered that acidic and alkaline extremes in the body cause the steady, low-oxygen environment that cancer needs to survive. Dr. Warburg reportedly produced cancer in forty-two species of animals simply by lowering their pH levels, causing an acidic environment and depriving their cells of oxygen. He proved that an acidic environment and low oxygen levels in the body can lead to disease.[1]

Foods in their raw form supply oxygen to the body. Cooking reduces oxygen. The best way to increase oxygen in our cells and ward off infection is to exercise and eat a diet high in raw, whole natural foods. Foods that are high in oxygen are leafy greens, raw fruits and vegetables.

Stress, negative thoughts, and emotions can also cause an imbalance in your body. Adrenalin reduces the flow of blood in vessels and inhibits oxygen from moving to body cells. Whether the stress is physical, mental, or emotional, you can do something about it. Go for walks, exercise moderately, socialize with friends, get a massage, read a good book, get professional help, meditate, use biofeedback, or get hypnotherapy. Do whatever it takes to remove stress and change negative thoughts and emotions. Look at my website for a meditation for releasing stress at www.janefalke. com/stress-release.

Most drugs, whether prescribed, over-the-counter, or recreational, produce unhealthy side-effects in the body. You can control your need for over-the-counter drugs, and possibly reduce or discontinue medications, simply by changing what you eat to whole natural foods and pure mineral rich water.

Pollutants come from our environment through the air we breathe and chemicals in the water we drink and bathe in. Pollutants also come from our homes and gardens, from pesticides used on our food, and from smoking tobacco products. Find ways to minimize or eliminate these pollutants in your environment.

Coffee, caffeinated tea, and soft drinks are stimulants. They are very addictive and toxic to the body. They dehydrate you and "steal" vitamins and minerals from your body. Cut down on them, and then give them up altogether. Eliminating them from your diet slowly prevents suffering from headaches and other symptoms of withdrawal. The more outside stimulation your body receives, the less energy you have!

Sustaining Health with Balanced Nutrition

Whether alcohol comes from hard liquor, beer, or wine, it is absorbed directly into the bloodstream from the small intestines. It gives you a direct hit of relaxation and calmness, and that's why it is addictive. It is also dehydrating to your body. Liquor is fermented, brewed, and turns into ethanol – a toxic poison. Wine is fermented and usually processed with sulfites that kill the natural enzymes in grapes. Your liver works overtime trying to filter out the toxins in these beverages. Cut down and then eliminate them.

Look at ways that you may be contributing to your health problems and make changes before it is too late. You can control many toxic conditions by changing your diet, making healthy lifestyle changes, and exercising. Taking these steps is much simpler than taking medications, having medical procedures, and suffering from illness and disease.

Chapter 9
A Chance for Change

Why Is It Hard to Change?

In order to experience change in your life, you have to initiate the change by changing a thought, belief, or habit. Habits are repeated behavior patterns. They become part of you even though you may not be aware of it. Soon they become part of your personality and belief system.

Family habits, traditions, and upbringing pattern our personal habits, beliefs, and behavior. We learn certain behaviors that become part of our being without noticing how these patterns continually affect our lives.

Sometimes we need a story to remind us that our lives are important. This message is traveling the internet and provides an opportunity to see things in a different light:

> An elderly Chinese woman had two large pots, each hung on the ends of a pole that she carried across the back of her neck. One of the pots had a crack in it while the other pot was perfect and always delivered a full portion of water. At the end of the long walks from the stream to the house, the cracked pot arrived only half full.

For a full two years the woman brought home only one and a half pots of water. Of course, the perfect pot was proud of its accomplishments. But the poor, cracked pot was ashamed of its own imperfection, and miserable about being able to do only half of what it had been made to do. After two years of what it perceived to be bitter failure, it spoke to the woman one day by the stream. "I am ashamed of myself because this crack in my side causes water to leak out all the way back to your house."

The old woman smiled. "Did you notice that there are flowers on your side of the path, but not on the other pot's side? That's because I have always known about your flaw, so I planted flower seeds on your side of the path, and every day while we walk back, you water them. For two years I have been able to pick these beautiful flowers to decorate the table. Without your being just the way you are, there would not be this beauty to grace the house."

Each of us has our own unique flaws. But it's the cracks and flaws we each have that make our lives together so very interesting and rewarding. Look for the good in everyone, including yourself. Let go of negative self-talk. Do not accept thoughts and feelings that beat you down. To help yourself in making diet and lifestyle changes, recognize and accept who and what you are right now. Then look at what you want. Wanting attracts opportunities, and doors start to open, offering more opportunities for change.

Change is a good thing. Life is always changing whether we want it to or not. Resisting change disrupts the flow of life, and you can become frustrated and angry when you try to control the flow of life and realize that you really can't control it. When you accept the flow of life, you can move forward with an attitude of anticipation.

But though you cannot control everything in your life, you can control your thoughts, choices, and decisions. When you make a decision about your life, you are choosing a course of action to follow. When I feel something holding me back, I use a meditation process to discover what it is and make productive decisions. If you would like help overcoming old habits and making positive changes, refer to my website, www.janefalke. com/changing-your-habit-patterns.

Here's my story:

When I was four years old, my mother took me to the barber and had my hair shaved off. She heard this would make my hair grow back thicker. I was embarrassed walking home and did not want anyone to see me that way. I made the decision that I would never stand out again. But this decision held me back. I was very shy. I did not speak much to anyone except my close family members. I never raised my hand in school. I avoided situations in which I had to speak in front of a group. I had a difficult time with social situations. It took me years to become more outgoing and move forward without so much fear of being judged as not good enough.

I did not remember this part of my childhood until I was about forty years old. It unfolded during meditation while I was working through my fear of public speaking. I asked my mother if it had actually happened, and she was surprised that I remembered it.

I did much of my personal growth work in meditation. I began to see myself as I wanted to be. I imagined myself speaking in public and speaking out in various situations. Over time I slowly opened up, and now I teach others to be healthy through visualization, meditation, yoga, and nutritional coaching.

You can make changes, too. Once you identify what you wish to accomplish, you can generate new thoughts, habits, and beliefs through repetition.

How to Make a Change

Life provides us with results and consequences from what we think and believe. Your thoughts create what is in your life rather than your being subject to the whims of life and other people. If you think negative thoughts about yourself, you are holding yourself in that place and attracting what you are thinking about. If you think positive, uplifting thoughts, you will attract more positive thoughts to you and be the cause of change in your life.

The Cleansing Program and The Maintenance Program comprise a fourteen-day plan to get you started toward your three-month goal of improved health. It begins with following a simple method of ensuring success as you change into a new, healthy you. When you know what you want, you can easily plan how to make it happen. The Three Principles of Success will help you make the change.

Principle #1 - Be Clear about What You Want

In order to be clear about what you want, you must know what you want. Think about the health goal you wish to accomplish over the next three months.

Eat Healthy. Be Healthy at Any Age.

Think about it as if you already have it. Write down a sentence describing what you want in the present tense. For example, "I am happy I weigh [xxx] pounds," or "I am happy I can wear my black pants again," or "I eat a nutritious diet and feel strong, energized, and healthy," or "I feel great that my digestion is efficient now that I eat healthier foods."

_____

_____

_____

It has taken time to get where you are today. Be practical about your expectations and goals. As you make changes in your habits and imagine already having your goal, you will eventually make changes in your overall health as well.

Principle #2 - Be Truthful about What You Can and Will Do

In order to accomplish your goal, you must be truthful about the commitments you can and will keep. You can be willing to do something, but not able to. And you can be able to do something, but not willing. When you are willing *and* able to commit to your plan, results are easily accomplished.

This principle is about making a plan that works for you. For instance, if your goal is to lose weight, what are the things you are able to do to accomplish this goal? If you are unable to go to a gym, think about what you are able to do for exercise. Is it going for a fast walk three days a week? Or doing stretching exercises every day? Start with what you can do. Later you can incorporate more to further your success.

After you list what you can do, ask yourself whether or not you are willing to do these things. We often say we will do something but don't do it. Then we feel badly. Continual failure can lead to feelings of worthlessness, hopelessness, and helplessness. This does not have to happen. Write down what you can and will do over the next fourteen days that will contribute to your three-month goal.

_____

_____

_____

Principle #3 – Be Responsible for the Outcome

Part One – Commitment

This principle asks you to be responsible for the result you want to accomplish – your goal. There are two parts to being responsible. The first part is committing to do your health plan for fourteen days, and then DOING IT. Give yourself the opportunity to see the change in your body and notice your attitude and changes in your confidence, self-worth, and health. By making a commitment to yourself to follow through on your plan, you are being responsible for the outcome of your health.

Are you willing and able to DO your health plan over the next fourteen days?
_____ Yes, I am!

Part Two – Assessing Your Progress

The second part of being responsible is evaluating the results of your actions. After you complete The Cleansing Program and The Maintenance Program, you can assess your progress.

Eat Healthy. Be Healthy at Any Age.

What worked? Look at what you did over the past fourteen days. Weigh yourself. Take measurements and pictures of your body again. Write down those things that worked so you will continue to do them:

_____

_____

_____

What could work better? One of the best ways to make changes for a better future is to evaluate the past without self-judgment. Perhaps you followed your plan but it was difficult. You may need to add more exercises or drink more pure water. By working on this ongoing plan, your next steps will be easier. Write down those things that could work better:

_____

_____

_____

Keep using these principles every week until you achieve your desired results. Knowing what you want and making a plan will help you achieve it faster than anything else.

PART II
Your Health Program

Eat Healthy. Be Healthy at Any Age.

As you learned in Part I, food can be detrimental to your health when you are unaware of how it is grown and manufactured. Currently the food industry does not focus on your overall health. It develops products for profits. This is why convenient and processed foods can be problematic to your health. The only way to control your health through food is to make healthy choices about what goes in your mouth. Choosing the right food is your solution to good health.

As you begin a healthy lifestyle change, it is important to eliminate accumulated toxins from past food choices and what you accrued through environmental pollutants. Part II addresses this subject by offering a complete program of cleansing your body and teaching you how to eat after The Cleansing Program. This strategy helps combat the vicious cycle of poor health and attain a healthy, ideal body through balanced nutrition and appropriate exercise.

Your Health Program begins with The Mini-Cleanse, then proceeds to The Cleansing Program and The Maintenance Program, and includes exercise. Afterward you will evaluate your results and develop your plan to continue eating healthy foods.

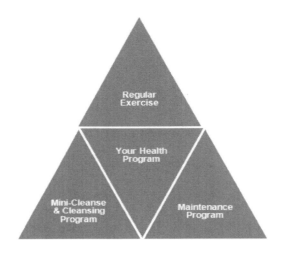

Nutritional Supplements

You may ask, "Should I take nutritional supplements?" The answer is yes and no. Yes, take nutritional supplements if you eat out regularly, eat processed foods, or eat conventionally grown foods. A good quality vitamin and mineral supplement once a day can be very helpful. Even so, you will not obtain all the nutrients, antioxidants, and phytonutrients needed for optimal health from supplements. They are manufactured products too complex to deliver the percentages of nutrients stated on the bottles. And many brands include stabilizers, anticaking agents, humectants, and emulsifiers as preservatives. Many people take extra supplements "just for good measure," but this is not cost effective. You eliminate what your body doesn't need in your urine, literally flushing money down the toilet.

No, don't take supplements if you are healthy, eat whole, natural, organically grown foods from sustainably managed farms, and don't eat processed foods stripped of their nutrient value. A large percentage of the ingredients in supplements are not absorbed by the body because they are synthetic. When you are giving the body what it needs by eating a balanced diet of whole, natural, plant-based foods, you are likely not to need additional supplements.

If you buy supplements, ask for a quality product without stabilizers. Several brands are pure. Health food stores usually offer some brands that don't use additives. Always look at the "other ingredients" listed on the label before buying, and ask questions if you don't understand the contents.

You may also ask, "Why can't I just eat the American diet and take nutritional supplements to get the nutrients I need?" Nutritional supplements supplement your diet. It's more difficult for the body to absorb the ingredients in supplements than it is to absorb the nutrients found naturally in foods. Whole foods supply the best nutritional benefits via easy-to-absorb nutrients in moderate amounts designed for your body by nature.

Locally Grown Foods

Locally grown foods are fresh because no time is wasted on shipping, and are grown during their natural growing season so they provide the highest nutrient value available. Various foods are available at the peak of their individual growing season, from early spring through late fall (and into the winter if you live in a southern climate), supplying various nutrients and flavors throughout the year.

The longer it takes food to get from the farm to your table, the fewer nutrients it contains. And the more transportation and fuel needed to ship it, the higher the price tag. Foods from foreign countries are not grown under US standards, and may contain pesticides banned in the US. By eating a variety of locally grown, whole, organic foods, you will be on your way to better health.

Science is continually discovering the ways the body uses micronutrients. There is a promising future for natural remedies and completely new ways to treat and cure diseases. By eating a balanced nutrient-filled diet, your body can have what it needs for good health now without waiting for science to prove that this is so.

Chapter 10
The Benefits of Regular Exercise

Our ancestors did not have the conveniences we have today. Their work entailed physical labor rather than sitting at a desk. They burned more calories than we do today, and ate meals that came from local farms and home gardens. Exercise was a natural part of their day.

Today much of our time is spent in front of our computers and driving our cars to and from work, errands, and shopping. Little energy is expended. We consume more food and exercise less. Consequently we are gaining weight, losing physical strength, and challenging our health.

But there are lots of ways to get the exercise our bodies need. We have fitness centers and home gyms with weights and machines to help gain and maintain our physical strength. Throughout our cities, exercise classes offer many options to suit our interests. With what is available, why is it that many people still do not exercise?

We have our reasons for not exercising: "I don't have time," "I don't enjoy it," "It's too hard," "I don't like to sweat." These reasons may be valid, but a lifetime of such reasons can result in muscular and skeletal problems. General body weaknesses come from lack of strength and flexibility. We see older people bent over with osteoporosis from bone and mineral loss, and with flabby arm and leg muscles from muscle wasting (loss). Low back issues are common due to lack of core strength. Physical inactivity can initiate many chronic ailments and pain.

Exercise helps boost metabolism – the total amount of energy your body burns over a specific time. Even if you lead a sedentary lifestyle, your body still needs to burn energy for breathing, beating your heart, cell and organ function, and thinking. The basal metabolic rate (BMR) is the minimum amount of energy needed to sustain life. BMR influences how rapidly food converts into energy. A slow BMR can cause weight gain and hormonal changes, which can lead to challenges in physical performance. A fast BMR can help burn calories and keep your body healthy like a finely tuned automobile.

You can improve your metabolism by eating smaller portions of food more often and performing activities that make you sweat, such as taking a sauna or exercising.

Exercise not only boosts your metabolism, but it is a sure way to lift your spirits. It improves your posture and increases your breathing capacity. It is the best way to keep your body structurally fit. Exercise should be fun, safe, and comfortable. Here are ten benefits of exercise:

- Strengthens and tones muscles
- Increases flexibility and balance
- Helps maintain bone mineral density
- Increases breathing capacity and energy

Your Health Program

- Moves toxins through the lymphatic system
- Relieves stress and depression
- Burns calories and helps control weight by raising metabolic rate
- Increases good (HDL) cholesterol, lowers total cholesterol
- Helps improve sleep
- Keeps the body structurally healthy

With these benefits, why not give exercise a try? If you are not actively exercising now, start out slowly. Invite a friend to join you for motivation and enjoyment. Pick out a workable time. Pick activities you enjoy and add more activities as you become stronger and more comfortable. You can join a gym and take classes to help you get started. This way you can learn what is best for your body and minimize injuries.

Start your exercise program with 15 to 30 minutes two days a week. Then increase it to three days a week. Vary what you do each day. For instance, one day you could take a yoga class or water aerobics, another day lift weights, and another day briskly walk. Here are some reasonable activities to get you started:

- Walking quickly for 1 to 2 miles
- Yoga for stretching and toning
- Water aerobics offered at many community pools
- Lift weights at home or at your local gym
- Chair aerobics
- Biking on level ground
- Active sports – running, throwing, moving fast
- Swimming
- Fast dancing, line dancing
- Moderate gardening – raking, trimming, and cleaning up
- You can also go to my website for a downloadable yoga practice: www.janefalke.com/inner-yoga

83

Eat Healthy. Be Healthy at Any Age.

After a few weeks or months, when you feel you are ready, pick up the pace of your chosen activities or add different ones. Do them longer by moving from 30 minutes to 45 or 60 minutes. Increase your days per week from three to four or five days a week. Increase your time or days per week slowly. Here are suggestions for more dynamic activities:

- Power yoga
- Martial arts
- Step aerobics or zumba
- Hiking
- Fast walking for 4 to 5 miles
- Running or jogging
- Biking up hills
- Swimming laps
- Tennis
- Weight training using heavier weights or stronger bands and machines

Strength training, also called weight and resistance training, is the best way to build muscle, prevent muscle wasting (loss), and strengthen bones. You want to improve every part of your body – arms, legs, chest, upper back, lower back, hips, buttocks, and abdominal muscles. Do these workouts at least three times a week. You will notice a big difference in your body strength as well as your attitude.

Aerobic exercise works your heart and lungs. It increases your heart rate, making it beat faster, which increases the amount of oxygen available to the muscles. Determine your maximum heart rate in order to reach the correct heart rate for you during aerobic exercise. Calculate your maximum heart rate by subtracting your age from 220. During aerobic exercise, achieve a target heart rate of 50 percent to 70 percent of your maximum heart rate. As an example, if you are 65 years old, 220 − 65 = 155. This is your maximum heart rate. Take 155 X 50% = 77 and 155 X 70% = 108. Your target heart rate is between 77 and 108.

During exercise, find your heart rate (pulse) by touching the artery in your wrist using the index and middle fingers of the opposite hand. Count how many beats during a 15-second period. Multiply this amount by 4 to reach your heart rate per minute. Increase or decrease your activity level to reach your target heart rate. Over time you can increase your target heart rate to 85 percent of your maximum heart rate for maximum benefit. You will know when you are ready for this increase.

Along with the benefits of exercise may come injuries. Do not overdo any type of exercise. Injuries will only take you backwards. Joints are the hardest hit during strength and aerobic activity. Protect your joints and yourself, and find the right balance for you.

Track your progress by using an exercise log. It can keep you motivated to continue your exercise program. It will also help you determine whether you need to alter your exercise program. Here is a sample daily exercise log you can use:

Date	Time of day	Activity	Goal to achieve	Achieved today	How you felt
3/12	8:00 a.m.	yoga	60 minutes	60 minutes	Energized
3/14	8:00 a.m.	fast walking	4 miles	3 miles	Great
3/16	8:00 a.m.	weight lifting	10 lb. weights	5 lb. weights	Stronger

If you have medical challenges, speak with your doctor before starting an exercise program. Your doctor should suggest the type of exercise that is right for you. There are many hospitals that offer fitness programs for patients with serious health conditions, or perhaps you need physical therapy before you can start a regular exercise program. Plan the activities you are willing and able to do.

Chapter 11
Why Cleanse the Internal Body?

The most effective way to begin healing and removing toxins from your body is with a cleanse. Internal cleansing is a holistic therapy that allows your body to heal itself naturally. It includes removing the debris that has built up in your body and providing the nutrients and raw materials – or building blocks – for repair and energy.

Here are some benefits of internal cleansing:

- Remove plaque and toxins
- Repair the small intestines
- Build healthy blood
- Clear congestion in the lymphatic system
- Relieve bloating and sluggishness
- Provide energy to your body
- Reduce fat and body weight
- Put a smile on your face

Everything we eat and drink goes to the small intestines where intestinal villi absorb nutrients, then moves into the bloodstream to feed these nutrients to your cells. Blood and lymphatic capillaries take back the fluids to further filter and detoxify them, and they are sent to the elimination organs – lungs, skin, kidneys, and colon – for excretion. This is the natural function of the body.

Eat Healthy. Be Healthy at Any Age.

However, damage can come to the intestinal villi by what we eat and drink. Such damage is mainly due to overconsumption of protein and ingestion of sugar and foods that metabolize to sugar. When protein breaks down, it forms strong acids including nitric, sulfuric, phosphoric, and uric acid that can burn holes in clothes, metal, and human cells. These acids can eventually break down the villi and make it more difficult to absorb nutrients.

Villi are finger-like projections on the inside walls of the small intestines. In the projections are blood and lymphatic vessels that absorb nutrients.

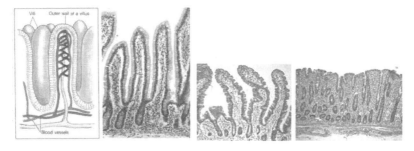

Blood Vessels   Healthy   Unhealthy, damaged Villi
  in Villi   Villi

Blood is considered a vital life force and the most important material of the human body. It transports nutrients, oxygen, hormones, and proteins to cells. Blood moves waste and carbon dioxide to the organs of elimination for disposal. You cannot live without your blood.

The most important food we can provide for our bodies to help build blood is chlorophyll, because the molecular structures of chlorophyll and red blood cells are almost identical. The primary difference is that chlorophyll has magnesium at its core to enhance photosynthesis, while blood has iron to utilize oxygen.

Eating more chlorophyll from green foods builds red blood cells and provides oxygen that helps rid the body of microorganisms – bacteria, yeast, fungus, molds, and viruses. These microorganisms cannot live in an oxygen filled environment.

During health challenges, your doctor will likely order blood tests to identify problem areas. These tests provide quantities of substances such as cholesterol and triglycerides in the blood. Your doctor can then appropriately diagnose and treat unhealthy conditions with medications, therapies, or surgery.

I am trained in live and dry blood analysis, a technique using a few drops of blood to identify the quality of the blood. Live blood shows the present condition of the blood. Dry blood shows the condition of the organ systems in the body. This technique does not diagnosis disease; it gathers information about health and nutritional needs to identify possible patterns of disorganization in the blood. From this analysis one can determine the potential effectiveness of certain methods or procedures and, if serious damage is revealed, medical advice can be sought.

Here is an example of live red blood cells (RBC):

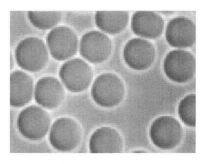 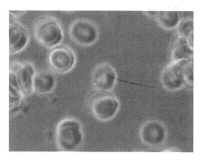

Healthy Live Blood
Evenly round RBCs Clean and clear fluid between

Unhealthy Live Blood
Some RBCs stuck together
Different sizes, white spots in the middle
Bacteria and fibrin in the plasma

Eat Healthy. Be Healthy at Any Age.

Blood can reveal imbalances due to a compromised pH (potential of hydrogen) level. Acidity or alkalinity is measured on a scale from one to fourteen. A pH value below seven is acidic, and above seven is alkaline. The blood must preserve a slightly alkaline pH range between 7.35 and 7.45 to keep the body healthy. Blood naturally seeks what it needs from the body to preserve this delicate range. Pulling alkaline minerals from the body leaves tissues acidic. Acidity is a big problem today because of the processed and refined foods consumed in the standard American diet.

The lymphatic system carries toxic wastes away from tissues, then out of the body. When this system is congested, wastes do not move out of the body and the pressure of the congestion causes waste to move back into the tissues, skin, and joints, causing further stress to the liver and chronic aches and pains. You can clear congestion in the lymphatic system through dietary changes, sweating during exercise, using a far infrared sauna, or having lymphatic massages. When wastes flow out of the body, nutrients can be absorbed and the body naturally heals itself.

An example of dry blood:

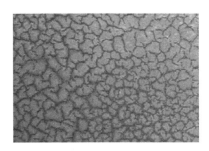 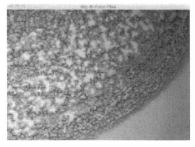

Healthy Dry Blood

Congested Lymphatic System shown in Dry Blood Analysis

Your Health Program

We experience imbalances and symptoms of disease every day. Low energy and fatigue, poor digestion, excess weight, unclear thinking, aches and pains, aging, and chronic disease are just some such symptoms of imbalance. To balance your health you must remove toxins from your body and alkalize your system. Alkaline materials come from clean water, oxygen, chlorophyll, minerals, alkaline foods, and balanced nutrition. Alkaline materials are what make new and healthy cells.

Detoxification and internal cleansing is a process. We take in toxins every day, and it takes time to remove them, heal the small intestines, and change the blood. Therefore it is important to cleanse and detoxify your body regularly – every three or four months.

Here are some of the results and comments from my clients who have gone through The Cleansing Program:

- Felt cleaned out
- Joints less stiff
- Less mucus
- Less nasal conjestion
- Did not feel hungry
- Lost appetite for sweets
- Invigorated
- Slept soundly
- Less pain
- Felt good – the way I want to feel again
- Didn't need my usual analgesics for arthritis or back pain
- Glad I did it
- Average weight loss 7.5 pounds
- Average loss of inches on body: 5.75"

Now that you have learned the importance of balanced nutrition and regular exercise, you can start Your Health Program.

Chapter 12
Preparing for Your Health Program

Before you begin Your Health Program there are some details to organize and items to buy. Here are some suggestions:

Clean Out Your Refrigerator, Freezer, and Pantry

There are so many reasons to remove foods that are not healthy for you. The obvious one has to do with your past eating habits. To help break these habits, get rid of junk foods, unhealthy snacks, aged herbs and spices, and refined, packaged, and canned foods that are out of date.

Equipment for Your Kitchen

The items listed below are great investments for your health. If you are on a tight budget, start with a blender and a juicer.

- Blender to pulverize and puree foods and make nut and seed milks, soups, sauces, and smoothies. High-speed blenders produce the best results

- Juicer to extract juice from pulp, leaving beneficial, absorbable nutrients
- Cheese cloth, fine strainer, or nut and juice bags for straining nut milks, seed milks, and juices
- Quart and pint canning jars with wide mouths for soaking, sprouting, and storing nuts, seeds, grains, and legumes
- Water – purified, filtered, reverse osmosis, or alkaline water to drink, add to recipes, and soak nuts and seeds

These make food preparation easy and fast:

- Food processor for chopping, grating, slicing, and making salad dressings
- Food saver provides longer shelf life for foods by taking the air out of canning jars and plastic vacuum-seal bags. When you purchase a food saver, get the canning-jar attachment
- Coffee grinder or mini-blender for grinding seeds, nuts, and dried herbs into powders and making quick salad dressings
- Dehydrator optimizes the nutrient value in foods through low temperatures. Use it to warm foods and make "meat" balls and loaves, burgers, muesli, cereals, crackers, and breads

Order the Cleansing Program Supplements

Go to www.janefalke.com/cleansing-package

Your Fourteen-Day Health Plan

Days One through Seven

- Take pictures of yourself – full body and a close-up of your face.

Eat Healthy. Be Healthy at Any Age.

- Take your body measurements, weigh yourself, and write down the numbers.
- Set your goal for the next three months.
  - Refer to Principle of Success #1 (see Chapter 9)
  - What do you want to accomplish?
- Make an appropriate plan for following through.
  - Refer to Principle of Success #2
  - What are you willing and able to do?
- Buy groceries for The Cleansing Program. A grocery list is included in an upcoming chapter.
- Wash your produce and put it away. Debbie Meyer™ Green Bags® are great for longer-lasting produce.
- Do The Cleansing Program for a minimum of seven days (10 to 14 days is better).

Days Eight through Fourteen

- Look over your menu plan, make out your grocery list, and buy groceries for The Maintenance Program.
- Wash your produce and put it away.
- Do The Maintenance Program for a minimum of seven days (longer is better)

Day Fifteen

- Take pictures of yourself – full body and face.
- Take your body measurements, weigh yourself, and write down the losses.
- Evaluate your results
  - Use Principle of Success #3
  - What worked?
  - What could work better?

Your Health Program

- Use the Three Principles of Success to make a new plan to continue The Maintenance Program for at least three months. When you see the results and experience the benefits, you will want to continue The Maintenance Program for a lifetime.

You have learned the importance of cleansing your body of toxins and providing it with nutrients. This is how to be healthy. There are many recipes and books about a plant-based diet available on the internet or in bookstores. You can go to my website for more recipes: http://www.janefalke.com/category/recipes/.

To your health! Enjoy the process!

Chapter 13
The Mini-Cleanse

Fast-paced lives usually include fast-food meals, prepackaged meals that you heat and eat, or regularly eating at restaurants. Convenience foods contain refined products and chemical additives that are toxic to our bodies. Toxins also come from air, water, cleaning supplies, building materials in our homes and workplaces, lotions, and many other substances in our environment. Toxins challenge our bodies' natural healing processes and sap our energy.

The liver detoxifies substances before they enter the bloodstream and move into the cells. When the liver is overwhelmed with too many toxins, they accumulate in the internal organs, cells, and tissues. Toxins can inhibit healthy body maintenance and recovery from unhealthy conditions, making us more sluggish, bloated, and fatigued. If you feel this way, you can bring balance to your body with the ultimate fast food that takes little time to prepare and offers a wealth of nutrition and healing powers: juice!

Benefits of Juicing

- Provides balanced nutrition
- Increases physical energy

Your Health Program

- Contributes to youthful skin and clear eyes
- Detoxifies the liver
- Supports a strong immune system

Juicing brings fresh, raw materials to your body for healing. Juiced vegetables and low-sugar fruits improve the function of the liver and the elimination organs by providing balanced nutrients that help remove accumulated toxic substances. They provide essential vitamins, minerals, antioxidants, phytonutrients, chlorophyll, enzymes, amino acids, purified water, and oxygen. The entire body then operates more efficiently with improved immune function and increased energy.

- Vitamins and minerals are essential building blocks for energy and body material.
- Antioxidants help boost the immune system by keeping free-radical damage from harming and aging the body.
- Phytonutrients are nature's medicines for maintaining health and preventing disease.
- Chlorophyll is an effective internal cleanser, blood builder, and energizer, and provides protein in the form of amino acids.
- Enzymes are complex proteins important to every chemical function of the body.
- Amino acids are building blocks of protein that form and repair bodily tissue.
- Purified water is essential to the body's mineral and electrolyte balance.
- Oxygen is necessary for every cell in the body. Without oxygen, cells die and microorganisms breed.

Consuming juiced foods rests the body from eating, chewing, and digesting macronutrients: carbohydrates, fats, and animal protein. Your body receives an abundant amount of easily absorbed micronutrients.

Eat Healthy. Be Healthy at Any Age.

Think of juices as providing your body with natural medicine. The nutrients go to work immediately, removing toxins and minimizing free-radical damage.

Many Ways to Use the Mini-Cleanse

- Three days before The Cleansing Program
- Three or more days anytime you feel bloated, uncomfortable, or have a cold or flu
- One day during the week or month to rest the digestive organs
- One or two meals any day
- As a snack or any time you are hungry

Some people should not shift their diets to fluids all at once. Check with your doctor before starting The Mini-Cleanse. You can reap the benefits by instead adding juice as a snack or to your meals rather than drinking tea, coffee, milk, and soft drinks.

How Much Juice Should You Drink?

Aim for at least four 16 to 20 ounce glasses of juice each day. If your energy is low during The Mini-Cleanse, or you feel hungry or have flu-like symptoms, drink more water and vegetable juice. This will aid in removal of toxins through the elimination organs.

Tips for Making Juice

- Buy organic produce to eliminate pesticide residue and genetically engineered foods.
- Wash and chop vegetables before juicing to fit into the juicer.
- Do not peel vegetables. Peels contain vital nutrients.

- Leave stems on greens and herbs.
- Mix hard and soft vegetables.
- Strain the foam from the juice before you drink it.
- You can double or triple the recipes, but keep the juice covered in the refrigerator or in a cold container to take with you for no more than twenty-four hours. If you have a food saver with a canning-jar attachment, use it to take out the air in the jar to save the vital nutrients for a longer period of time.
- All the juicing recipes make sixteen to twenty ounces of high potency, alkaline juice.
- If your juicer does not make at least sixteen ounces, run the pulp through the juicer again or add alkaline water to the juice.
- Chew the juice a few times to active the enzymes in your saliva for better absorption.
- Fresh turmeric root, if you can find it, cleanses the liver and fights cancer. Add ½ inch to each juicing recipe or use 1 teaspoon of the powdered version.

Suggested Three-Day Menu Plan for the Mini-Cleanse (Recipes are in Part III)	
Day One	
Juice 1	The Energizer
Juice 2	Mineral Power
Juice 3	A Glass of Salad
Juice 4	Green Power Juice
Day Two	
Juice 1	Popeye Power
Juice 2	V8 Tomato Juice

Eat Healthy. Be Healthy at Any Age.

Juice 3	Cucumber Salad in a Glass
Juice 4	Mean Green Juice
Day Three	
Juice 1	Immune Booster
Juice 2	Alkaline Power
Juice 3	Liver Cleanse
Juice 4	Triple C

Suggested Grocery List for The Mini-Cleanse	
2 lemons	3 heads celery
Fresh mint	6 roma tomatoes
1 garlic bulb	10 cucumbers
6 inches fresh turmeric root or powder	1 pound baby spinach
5 inches fresh ginger root	1 bunch romaine lettuce
2 bunches parsley	2 bunches kale
1 bunch green onions	1 head green cabbage
1 bunch radishes	1 bunch collard greens
2 small beets	4 green apples
2 red bell peppers	cayenne pepper
5 pounds carrots	

You can use The Mini-Cleanse anytime. It is not part of the fourteen-day health plan, but you can use it prior to starting The Cleansing Program if you choose.

Chapter 14
The Cleansing Program

Your fourteen-day health plan begins with seven days of The Cleansing Program. If you have health challenges, using The Cleansing Program for three or more weeks can be very effective for greater detoxification and improvement of your health.

This program is not a fast. It consists of the following:

- Blended smoothies
- Pureed soups
- Raw salads
- Essential fats and oils
- Nutritional supplements
- Alkaline water
- Lymphatic massage, far infrared saunas, and exercise
- Colon irrigation or enemas

Freshly juiced green vegetable smoothies and soups supply energy for the body which is easily utilized because no energy is expended for digestion. Eat one or two smoothies or bowls of soup at each meal, or more if you are hungry.

Essential fats – Add high-quality seeds to your smoothies and soups. Use hemp seeds (high in protein), ground flax seeds (high in fiber), or chia seeds (high in omega-3 fatty acids). If you do not have a high-speed blender like the Vitamix, use hemp oil, flax seed oil, or chia seed oil. Avocados give smoothies and soups a smooth texture and provide healthy monounsaturated fats.

Nutritional supplements – The supplements, The Cleansing Program Guide and The Maintenance Program Guide include every thing you will need to follow the program for a week and even longer. They will help make your cleanse and lifestyle change easy. In addition to what is offered in this book, the guides include a daily supplement schedule, pH chart for seven days, measurement and weight chart, and offers ideas on what to do as you continue eating healthy whole, natural foods after The Cleanse. The nutritional supplements and guides are on my website. Go to: http://www.janefalke. com/store/cleansing-supplements/

Alkaline water – It is important to drink a lot of water to help flush acids and toxins from your body. While on The Cleansing Program, drink one quart for every thirty pounds of body weight. If you weigh 150 pounds, drink five quarts per day. Build up to this amount. Use purified water, water filtered using reverse osmosis, or bottled water with added minerals and without sugar. Add pH drops to increase oxygen and alkalinity.

The lymphatic system is a major elimination system of the body, carrying toxic wastes away from tissues and out of the body. When this system is congested, wastes do not move out of the body and the pressure of the congestion causes wastes to move back into the tissues, skin, and joints, causing further stress to the liver. Toxins are moved out of the body through sweating and moving the muscles. Once the flow is re-established, the body can absorb and benefit from the nutrients provided and heal itself.

- **Lymphatic massage** is a gentle form of massage that stimulates the lymphatic system to improve metabolism, promote the removal of toxins and wastes from the body, and encourage a healthy immune system. Schedule two or three lymphatic massages during The Cleansing Program. Most massage therapists do lymphatic massage.
- **Far infrared saunas** provide a comfortable and relaxing experience with a wide array of therapeutic benefits. These saunas have 40 percent cooler temperatures than traditional saunas (110-130 F vs. 180-210 F in standard saunas). Heat causes toxins to be released from cells. It is easier to breathe during such a sauna because of the gentle, soothing heat. It has deeper heat penetration – up to three inches into the body. It makes you sweat two to three times more than standard saunas. Since sweat is manufactured from the lymph fluid, toxins present in the lymph fluid exit the body through the sweat. It is non-fatiguing, burns calories, and you lose weight, not just water. You can receive all these benefits while reading or relaxing. Drink a lot of alkaline water while you are in the sauna.
  During The Cleansing Program you can take a sauna every day, or at least three times a week, working your way up to 35 or 40 minutes each time. Some health clubs and day spas offer far infrared saunas for an extra charge.
- **Exercise** is not only important in building muscles and strong bones and toning the body, it also gives you the opportunity to sweat. Sweating unclogs the skin and lymphatic system. You can exercise three to five times a week at a fitness center or you can walk briskly. For those who are not able to exercise because of health issues or extreme overweight, you can use a rebounder

– a mini-trampoline – to move toxins out of the lymphatic system. The important thing is to keep your body moving.

- **Colonic irrigation and enemas** – Flushing the colon cleanses the bowels. It helps move out solidified fecal matter, waste products, toxins, and parasites. Since colonic irrigation gets rid of unwanted waste, people who undergo this therapy start feeling healthier and lighter immediately. During The Cleansing Program, have at least three colonics or give yourself enemas daily. You can locate a certified colon therapist in the yellow pages of your telephone book or search the internet.

Detoxification Side Effects

Not everyone goes through detox symptoms, but it can happen. During cleansing, toxins are dumped into the blood to be removed from the body. This can result in feeling worse before you feel better. Some detox symptoms are nausea, dizziness, headaches, fatigue, runny nose, skin irritations, and emotional issues. These flu-like symptoms are sometimes called a "healing crisis." It's a good sign! It shows that the cleansing process is effective and toxins are being expelled from the body and eliminated through wastes, mucus, etc.

The most important thing to do if you exhibit these symptoms is hydrate your body further with alkaline water and green juices. This allows toxins to exit the body and helps decrease discomfort. If detox symptoms get too uncomfortable or you feel you cannot function effectively, eat a salad with lemon juice and olive oil, eat soups without pureeing them, or eat some steamed broccoli or sautéed greens. This will slow down detoxification. But **don't give up!** Cleansing will put you years ahead in the healing process.

Other Things to Do during the Cleansing Program

Epsom salts or baking soda (aluminum free) baths

Stress can drain the body of magnesium, and Epsom salts contain magnesium sulfate. Baking soda contains sodium bicarbonate, an important mineral for the body. When salts and baking soda are dissolved in hot bath water, the minerals can be absorbed through the skin and replenish minerals in the body. The salts draw toxins from the body, sedate the nervous system, reduce swelling, relax muscles, and create a feeling of calm and relaxation. Take a hot bath every day with one cup Epsom salts and one cup baking soda.

Testing urine and saliva

Urine and saliva pH tests show how many minerals are in your body tissues. When you test your urine, it shows the pH, or alkalinity/acidity, of your tissues. When you test your saliva, it shows the pH of alkaline reserves – or lack of them – in the body. The time of day when you are most acidic is 2:00 a.m. in the morning, and you are most alkaline at 2:00 p.m. in the afternoon (if you work at night and sleep during the day, reverse these times). During the sleep cycle, your body is cleaning house, removing wastes, and repairing and replenishing your body as needed. Hence more acid load is in the urine during this time and is eliminated in the first urine of the day. The second urine of the day is a better indicator of acid/alkaline balance.

Eat Healthy. Be Healthy at Any Age.

Test your urine and saliva with pH strips. Test your saliva first thing in the morning before you do anything, and test your second urine of the morning. As soon as practical after 2:00 p.m. in the afternoon, test your saliva and urine. Before you go to bed, test your saliva and your last urine of the day. Urine should be tested mid-stream. Saliva should be tested by gathering up saliva on your tongue and placing the strip in the pool of saliva. Hold the wet strip to the color chart and write down the correlating number on the chart provided in The Cleansing Program Guide. You are aiming to maintain an alkalinity of 7.4 or greater.

Foods to Omit during the Cleansing Program

- coffee, caffeinated tea, alcohol, wine, beer, soda, mineral water
- vinegar of any kind – it promotes yeast growth
- fermented foods (soy sauce (except Bragg® Liquid Aminos™), yogurt, sauerkraut, etc.) – also promote yeast growth
- products with yeast (many canned and packaged foods contain yeast)
- sugar and artificial sugar (stevia is okay)
- all animal protein (anything from an animal – dairy products, cheese, eggs, meat, fish, chicken, turkey, pork, lamb, etc.)
- grains and products made with grains (rice, bread, pasta, crackers, dessert, flour, etc.)
- legumes and beans
- starchy vegetables (corn, beets, potatoes, yams, root vegetables, etc.)
- all fruit except non-sweet fruits such as lemons, limes, avocados, cucumbers, tomatoes)
- mushrooms – they are a fungus
- all packaged and processed foods (these are not

natural whole foods (except Pacific, Imagine, or Trader Joe's brands of vegetable broth, and unsweetened almond milk))

Tips

- Because you are blending your smoothies and soups, you can chop all the vegetables roughly. No knife skills are required for these recipes.
- When preparing meals, read over the complete recipe, take out all the ingredients and necessary kitchen tools, wash the vegetables (if you haven't already prepared and stored them), and then make the recipe.
- Add ginger, garlic, onions, fresh herbs, or non-starchy vegetables for more flavor, antioxidants, and phytonutrients.
- Add cayenne pepper to smoothies and soups to give them more zip. Cayenne is cleansing and alkalizing.
- Many of the soup recipes make three or four servings so you can have them available for several meals.
- When away from home, go to a juice bar and order two large green vegetable juices – one for lunch and one for dinner or a snack.
- You may have as much of the smoothies, juices, and soups you want.
- Use the juice recipes provided in The Mini-Cleanse for any meal or as a quick pick-me-up when you feel sluggish.
- You can use packaged organic creamed coconut and water (1 package creamed coconut blended with 3 cups water) in place of one Thai coconut. (See Appendix 4: Resource Guide for where to buy creamed coconut.)

Eat Healthy. Be Healthy at Any Age.

Suggested Seven-Day Cleansing Program Menu Plan (Recipes are in Part III)	
Day One	
Breakfast	The Energy Drink
Lunch	Cucumber Avocado Soup
Dinner	Celery Cauliflower Soup
Snack	½ to 1 cup Coconut Almond Milkshake
Day Two	
Breakfast	The Energy Drink, Too
Lunch	Large salad with mixed raw vegetables, chew to a liquid before swallowing
Dinner	No Tortilla Soup
Snack	1 cup Flavored Almond Milk
Day Three	
Breakfast	Green Coconut Smoothie
Lunch	Large salad with mixed raw vegetables, chew to a liquid before swallowing
Dinner	Celery Cauliflower Soup
Snack	drink the saved coconut water from your morning smoothie
Day Four	
Breakfast	The Energy Drink
Lunch	Large salad with mixed raw vegetables, chew to a liquid before swallowing
Dinner	No Tortilla Soup
Snack	½ to 1 cup Coconut Almond Milkshake

Your Health Program

Day Five	
Breakfast	The Energy Drink, Too
Lunch	Large salad with mixed raw vegetables, chew to a liquid before swallowing
Dinner	Creamy Broccoli Soup
Snack	1 cup Flavored Almond Milk

Day Six	
Breakfast	Green Coconut Smoothie
Lunch	Large salad with mixed raw vegetables, chew to a liquid before swallowing
Dinner	Rich Tomato Soup
Snack	Guacamole

Day Seven	
Breakfast	The Energy Drink
Lunch	Large salad with mixed raw vegetables, chew to a liquid before swallowing
Dinner	Creamy Broccoli Soup
Snack	1 avocado with sea salt and dash of cayenne pepper

Eat Healthy. Be Healthy at Any Age.

Grocery List for One Person	
Food	**Staples (you may already have these)**
3 cups raw almonds	sea salt
5 cucumbers	cayenne pepper
6 avocados	flax, hemp, or chia seeds or their oils
1 bunch kale	vanilla – Frontier brand (alcohol free)
1 lb. baby spinach	stevia – powdered or liquid drops
3-4 lemons or limes	coconut oil (use this for cooking)
2 Thai coconuts or 2 pkgs. organic creamed coconut	olive oil (drizzle on soups when serving)
1 head cauliflower	2 cartons vegetable broth (4 cups each)
2 pints cherry tomatoes	(Imagine, Pacific, and Trader Joe's
1 pkg. fresh mint leaves or	do not have yeast in them)
1 garlic bulb	mint extract (no alcohol)
2 inches fresh ginger	sun-dried tomatoes (not bottled)
1 bunch parsley	garlic granules
2 yellow onions	dried basil, oregano, thyme
3 lg. roma tomatoes brands	
2 jalapeno peppers	
1 bunch cilantro	
2 heads celery	
1 bunch carrots	
1 large head broccoli with stems	

Do The Cleansing Program for at least seven days, then do The Maintenance Program for a minimum of seven days. After you have evaluated your progress, continue with The Maintenance Program for a total of three months or until you have reached your health goals. By this time you will have changed many dietary habits and become much healthier. Continue eating whole, plant-based, alkaline foods as a lifestyle choice for your health.

110

Chapter 15
The Maintenance Program

After The Cleansing Program

The Maintenance Program is done for a minimum of seven days. The point is to eat healthy foods, not be on a diet. It teaches you how to use plant-based, alkaline foods and supports your body with continual internal cleansing and balanced nutrition through an abundance of healthy, whole, natural foods.

Warning

When you complete The Cleansing Program, please don't go back to a diet of mostly acidic foods or stop drinking your alkaline water. You will defeat the purpose of The Cleansing Program – ridding your body of toxins – and create once again an environment for unhealthy toxins in your body. Remember, a toxic, acidic internal environment provides the perfect breeding ground for microorganisms to multiply and eventually cause chronic disease.

Continue drinking alkaline water each day. You can drink the amount suggested in The Cleansing Program or drink one quart per day for every fifty pounds of your weight. More is better, because you still want to flush toxins from your body every day. Alkaline foods and alkaline water will keep you moving in the direction of healing the small intestines and bowels.

Speaking of bowels – most people think it is good and normal to have one bowel movement a day. This is truly not often enough. You eat at least three times a day; how about three bowel movements a day? If you can't do this on your own, take the Colon Cleanse capsules until you reach two or three movements a day.

Complex Carbohydrates

After The Cleansing Program, eat raw and lightly cooked or steamed vegetables such as steamed broccoli, green beans, and asparagus, and salads with lemon or olive-oil-based dressings. Slowly add complex carbohydrates back into your meals, but no more than 25% of your plate. You may add a serving per meal of peas, winter squash, sweet potato, pumpkin, split pea soup, or garbanzo beans or other legumes. Whole grains should be millet, spelt, buckwheat, quinoa, brown rice, and wheat, as long as they are free of sugar, honey, maple syrup, brown rice syrup, yeast, or any other addictive substance. Buckwheat, millet, quinoa, and spelt are the best, as they are not mucus-forming.

Exercising

Keep exercising. In addition to building muscle, strengthening bones, and moving the lymphatic system, exercise helps relieve stress and depression. After exercising, the "feel good" hormones serotonin and dopamine help change your attitude and lift your spirits.

Staying Balanced

The body preserves health when the cells are healthy. They multiply. An unhealthy cell greatly influences how the body functions. Toxic wastes are acidic and can poison and cause your cells to die.

We see the effects of balancing pH in a swimming pool. The pH of the water needs to be monitored, and adding proper chemicals prevents algae from growing. This applies to the pH of our bodies as well. We need to monitor the pH of our bodies, too.

Balance means your urine and saliva tests at 7.4 pH or above in the a.m. and p.m., every day. It also means you are at your ideal weight. If you are overweight, you should continue to free your body of acidic waste. Use the 75/25 rule (explained below) and keep your alkaline ratio as high as possible while losing weight, cleansing, and healing. Urine and saliva measurement are your benchmarks. If your pH strip shows lower than 7.4, take bicarbonate capsules immediately, and eat a higher percentage of alkaline foods.

Alkaline foods are those that contain large amounts of calcium, magnesium, sodium, and potassium. Most low-sugar fruits, greens, and vegetables, and some seeds, are alkaline. Acidic foods are those that contain phosphorus, chlorine, and sulfur. Your body needs these acidic minerals, but in small amounts. Meat; fish; poultry; legumes, seeds, and most nuts; grains; some fruits; and overcooked foods are acid-forming. Eating a nutrient-rich diet of alkaline foods and excluding refined and processed foods, and sugar results in a better pH balance in your body.

It is important to focus on eating a greater percentage of foods from alkaline foods – at least 75% – and no more than 25% from acidic foods. This is an easy ratio to remember and simplifies your food choices while you are learning which foods are alkaline and which are acidic or acid-forming. It is important to vary your foods from meal to meal and day to day to obtain the maximum amount of nutrients for good health.

Examples of Food Choices and Percentages

Breakfast: A green smoothie is a 100% alkaline meal. If you add a slice of toast made from Manna brand bread (your 25% acidic food portion) with raw almond butter, it fits the 75/25 rule.

Lunch: A large green salad with vegetables and alkaline dressing is a 100% alkaline meal. If you add one sprouted whole wheat tortilla with hummus, it fits the 75/25 rule.

Dinner: A large portion of vegetables and a dinner salad is a 100% alkaline meal. If you add 1/2 to 3/4 cup brown rice, it fits the 75/25 rule.

Animal Protein

I realize many people do not know how to eat or what to eat without animal protein in their diet. I do not recommend food from animals, but it is a personal choice. Here is why I don't eat animal products:

Commercially manufactured animals – common animal proteins such as beef, pork, lamb, chicken, and turkey that you find at the grocery store – are not fed a natural diet. In the first few months of life a cow is grazed on farm lands. Then it is shipped to a feedlot and fed a diet that fattens it up. This is where problems begin.

All these food animals – not only cows – are given corn, soy products, grains, refined oils, and hormones

114

to make them fatten up, which are not natural to their diets. Most of their diet consists of genetically modified (GM) products grown with the pesticides and herbicides discussed above. These are unnatural not only to the animals' diets, but to our diets, too. When you eat the animal muscle, you also ingest what has made that muscle – their food. Those GM foods, pesticides, antibiotics, hormones, and unhealthy oils become part of you. When you eat their diet – corn, soy, grains, processed oils – you get fat, too.

Feedlots and pens are devastating to animals. They are forced to live in their urine and feces, causing them to breathe and stand in many pollutants. They are given antibiotics to keep them disease-free. Can you imagine the stress they live under and the stress they experience when they go to the slaughterhouse? Stress releases harmful chemicals that remain in their flesh, which you will eat.

In addition to what is involved in manufacturing food animals, all animal protein, including dairy products, eggs, chicken, turkey, beef, pork, lamb, and fish, is naturally acidic. It is difficult to digest and congests the small and large intestines with hard-to-break-down protein particles. We have a major problem with constipation in the United States, and this undigested protein containing no fiber is a root cause.

Range-fed Animals

Grass- and range-fed animal products with very low levels of saturated fats and high concentrations of good omega-3 oils are available to us. They are more expensive, but they are a healthier alternative to eating manufactured animals. If you choose to eat animal protein, eat grass-fed or range-fed animals, but stay away from by-products such as cheese, milk, butter, and eggs. When you eat these, include them in the 25% acidic portion of your meal, and add lots of non-starchy vegetables. Other acidic foods like brown rice, beans, whole wheat pasta, legumes, and starchy vegetables are better choices for your 25% portion.

The Ancestral or Paleolithic Diet

The diet of our ancestors consisted mostly of meat and vegetables, with some fruits, nuts, and seeds. Dairy products were ingested in only a few cultures. This diet was healthy in the days when there were no feedlots, food industry, groceries stores, pesticides, or added hormones. Animals naturally grazed on healthy land. Vegetables were foraged on untreated and unpolluted lands. Organic foods were what the Earth provided naturally. This is not what we eat today. Animal foods are unhealthy options for required protein intake. We can get enough protein from the garden, and these are natural foods.

Dairy Products

Dairy products are high in saturated fats and the most mucus-forming foods on the planet. They cause a filmy congestion in your nose, mouth, throat, lungs, and digestive system. Mucus is a good thing when you are acidic. It is a protective coating that keeps the acids from burning holes in your cells, tissues, and organs. But mucus buildup, over time, can cause a multitude of illnesses. Do you have asthma? If you omit dairy products from your diet, you will no longer live with congestion or need mucus to save your life. You will not have to regularly blow your nose, cough, or clear your throat. Stay away from animal byproducts such as eggs, cheese, milk, butter, yogurt, and ice cream. They are breeding grounds for yeast, and can cause inflammation and congestion.

Wild-caught Fish

Fresh, wild-caught fish contains healthy fat with lower acidity than other animals, and can be part of The Maintenance Program on occasion. But because fish is known to contain mercury from contaminated waters, smaller wild-caught fish is your best choice. Large fish have more time to live in their environment, so contain greater quantities of pollutants. The US Environmental Protection Agency set guidelines in 2011 for fish consumption based on mercury levels, and reported that salmon, shrimp, clams, oysters, tilapia, scallops, catfish, and flounder have the lowest mercury levels. However, shellfish contain higher levels of cholesterol than fish that swim, and are not recommended. If you eat fish, choose fresh-water fish, because there are fewer pollutants in fresh water than in sea water, make it no more than 25% of your meal, and take bicarbonate capsules to help overcome the acidity.

Medications

When you begin to eat healthier, alkaline-forming foods, the chemistry in your body fluids changes and becomes more alkaline. Alkaline body fluids help repair and build a healthier body. As you continue The Maintenance Program, you may have to adjust the dose of medications you take downward from time to time, or eventually eliminate them altogether. *Work with your doctor*. Keep taking your medications until your doctor advises you differently.

Chewing Your Food

The Cleansing Program includes mostly blended foods because the process of breaking down the foods is already done for you, conserving the energy in the body for other things – healing and repairing. So it makes sense to continue to ingest blended foods. You do that by chewing your food well. Chew all the food in your mouth thirty to fifty times until it is liquid before you swallow. This is a good habit to develop because you feel full sooner and more easily avoid overeating.

The Maintenance Program Begins Now

Take baby steps to insure your success. You are learning a new way of thinking and preparing food. It can be a lot to learn all at once. In the weeks to come The Maintenance Program will be easier to follow as you become more familiar with the program, what foods to buy, and how to organize your time in the kitchen. You are developing new habits, which takes time. Baby steps equals success in your health and energy level, and you will soon feel better about yourself.

Tips to Save Time

Prepare a menu for breakfast, lunch, dinner, and snacks similar to the suggested menu in The Cleansing Program (see the suggested menu below). Exchange your favorite vegetable and herb ingredients in the recipes below using the lists in Appendix 3. It may seem time-consuming or cumbersome to prepare your meals. Here are some simple ways to save time:

- When on the run, take a storage bag with chopped veggies, sprouts, cherry tomatoes, nuts, seeds, or baked tofu to snack on. Planning ahead this way helps when you are faced with eating out.

- Most restaurants are happy to substitute extra veggies for meat or a starch. Try stir-fried dishes with steamed brown rice or have a spinach salad with veggies.
- Carry a small bottle of olive oil to use for dressing. You can ask for a few wedges of lime or lemon, or make your own dressing and carry it with you when you go out for a meal. Chinese, Thai, and Indian restaurants offer vegetarian and vegan meals.
- When you are at home, prepare things ahead of time. Make a big salad of mixed lettuces at the beginning of the week. Store it in an airtight container with paper towels lining the bottom to keep moisture and gasses naturally expelled from the vegetables from spoiling your greens.
- Wash and dry your vegetables, chop them, and keep them in sealed containers in the refrigerator ready to add to your salad at the last minute. There are many food processors and small hand-held choppers available to make salad preparation more convenient.
- Make several salad dressings ahead. They will last about ten days in the refrigerator.
- Soak almonds overnight to make Fresh Almond Milk for the next four days.
- Soak nuts and seeds overnight to make trail mix or seasoned seeds (see recipes) in larger amounts to use as needed.
- Make large batches of Sprouted Whole Wheat Tortilla Chips or Savory Seed Crackers. They will keep in the pantry for a month.
- Peel garlic cloves, mince, and cover with olive oil. Refrigerate in a glass jar for use in the recipes.
- Make pesto sauce, cover with olive oil, and freeze in small jars.

Eat Healthy. Be Healthy at Any Age.

Below is a suggested menu plan for the seven days of The Maintenance Program. Recipes for this menu plan follow in Part III. Depending on the time of year and your tastes, exchange other recipes for the ones below following the 75/25 rule and using plant-based, whole, natural foods.

Suggested Seven-Day Maintenance Program Menu Plan (Recipes are in Part III)	
Day One	
Breakfast	Lemon Tea, Breakfast Quinoa with Berries and Almonds
Lunch	Chopped Salad with Lemongrette Dressing
Main Meal	Brown Rice Bowl with Marinated Tofu and Vegetables Home-Style Carrot Salad
Snack	Spelt Puffed Crackers with Almond Butter
Drinks	Alkaline water, 3 to 4 quarts, 8 ounces fresh vegetable juice
Day Two	
Breakfast	Lemon Tea, Berry Smoothie, Toasted Manna Bread with Almond Butter
Lunch	Spinach Salad
Main Meal	Moroccan Vegetable Stew, Cucumber Salad
Snack	Sprouted Whole Wheat Tortilla Chips with Guacamole
Drinks	Alkaline water, 3 to 4 quarts, 8 ounces fresh vegetable juice
Day Three	
Breakfast	Lemon Tea, ½ grapefruit Creamy Buckwheat Cereal with Cinnamon, Vanilla, and Almonds
Lunch	Sweet and Spicy Kale Salad with Savory Seed Crackers
Main Meal	Pasta Prima Vera, Caesar Salad
Snack	Red peppers, zucchini, cucumber with Ranch Dressing
Drinks	Alkaline water, 3 to 4 quarts, 8 ounces fresh vegetable juice

Your Health Program

Day Four	
Breakfast	Lemon Tea, ½ grapefruit, Millet Porridge with Berries
Lunch	Tostada Salad
Main Meal	Gazpacho Soup, Mixed Green Salad with Lemongrette Dressing
Snack	Savory Seed Crackers with Guacamole
Drinks	Alkaline water, 3 to 4 quarts, 8 ounces fresh vegetable juice

Day Five	
Breakfast	Lemon Tea, Broccoli, Tomato, and Avocados
Lunch	Garden Wrap with Sweet Korean Dipping Sauce
Main Meal	Sesame Tofu with Spinach, Kale Slaw
Snack	Celery stalks with almond butter
Drinks	Alkaline water, 3 to 4 quarts, 8 ounces fresh vegetable juice

Day Six	
Breakfast	Lemon Tea, ½ grapefruit Creamy Brown Rice with Cinnamon, Vanilla, and Almonds
Lunch	Asparagus Salad with Mustard Dressing
Main Meal	Udon Noodles with Steam-Fried Vegetables Dinner Salad with your choice of dressing
Snack	Cherry tomatoes and carrot and celery sticks with Ranch Dressing
Drinks	Alkaline water, 3 to 4 quarts, 8 ounces fresh vegetable juice

Day Seven	
Breakfast	Lemon Tea, Scrambled Tofu with Spinach
Lunch	Asian Slaw with Wasabi Dressing
Main Meal	Vegetables in Parchment, Three Bean Salad
Snack	Sprouted Whole Wheat Tortilla Chips with Salsa
Drinks	Alkaline water, 3 to 4 quarts, 8 ounces fresh vegetable juice

Eat Healthy. Be Healthy at Any Age.

Set aside some time to prepare the following recipes in advance for the week:

Lemongrette Dressing
Herb Dressing To Go
Ranch Dressing
Caesar Dressing
Fresh Almond Milk

For snacks, cut up vegetables to dip in the dressings – red pepper, zucchini, cucumbers, carrots, and celery. Pack them in airtight containers and refrigerate. Make the following snacks in advance to eat as needed. Pack them in airtight containers and store them in your pantry:

Sprouted Whole Wheat Tortilla Chips
Savory Seed Crackers
Healthy Trail Mix

Chapter 16
Summary

Reseachers are discovering that unhealthy conditions in our bodies come from free-radical damage. As mentioned earlier, free radicals are generated when normal chemical activity in the body converts substances into energy. Environmental pollutants, tobacco smoke, alcohol, stress, pesticides, and food additives are some of the things that cause free radicals to overpopulate and produce damage in our bodies. This damage manifests as aging and chronic disease, and can cause early death from disease.

Accumulated toxins and acid from sugar, refined carbohydrates, processed foods, unhealthy fats, and manufactured animal products also contribute to free-radical damage. A diet rich in antioxidant, phytonutrient, plant-based, alkaline foods, and cleansing your body regularly, can counteract this damage.

You might be saying, "But I'll miss all the wonderful foods I grew up with. What about my grandma's recipe for lasagna with meat sauce that's such a favorite with my family? Or a hamburger and fries once in a while? And somtimes a bowl of ice cream just makes me feel good inside." You can enjoy these things, but make grandma's recipe with whole wheat or brown rice pasta, and marinara sauce without the meat but with added vegetables; replace beef burgers with veggie burgers or grilled vegetables, bake your fries in the oven instead of in refined oil, use a healthy whole-grain bun, and try sweet potatoes instead of russets; ice cream can be made with pureed frozen fruit instead of milk, sugar, and added chemicals. When you adapt recipes and adapt your attitude, your body adapts to feeling good and being healthy.

Remember the discussion about the habits of your taste buds in Chapter 2? Your taste buds will adapt to new recipes, too. When you use the recipes in this book, your tastes will change and you will no longer crave the added chemicals and artificial flavors of processed foods. You will actually prefer foods as nature intended them to be eaten – whole and healthy.

Going back to your old eating habits is no different from quitting smoking for a while, then having "just one puff" – you are addicted again! Or quitting drinking alcohol, then having "just one drink" – you are back to your old habit again! When you have removed beef from your diet, and have a steak because you are out with family or friends for a special occasion – you will be back to wanting it again, thinking, "Oh, just once won't hurt me." But you will have filled your body with acids, and they will challenge your body cells and start the cycle of imbalance all over again.

Your old eating habits caused your energy level to be low, your body to feel bloated and uncomfortable, and the pain of chronic health conditions. Unhealthy habits give you an unhealthy body and an unhealthy life. Commit to your health and stick with your plan. When you are challenged or tempted, remove yourself from the situation as soon as you can.

If I'm going out for a social engagement, I eat before I leave. Then I can pick and choose from what is being offered without letting hunger get the better of me. Restaurants now offer many healthy choices. One way around difficult menus is to order several plant-based side dishes rather than a main course. And many restaurants are willing to prepare something special for you. Just ask!

I've offered Four Essential Steps to Good Health in this book: commitment to your health, cleansing the internal body, balanced nutrition, and exercise. There are two programs for cleansing the body – The Mini-Cleanse and The Cleansing Program; The Maintenance Program, which furnishes balanced nutrition and suggestions for exercise; and the Three Principles of Success to help keep you on target with your commitment to health – not to mention the great recipes. The time is NOW to apply these health-promoting concepts as solutions to the chronic unhealthy conditions that are so prevelant in our society today.

Life is meant to be enjoyed without suffering or pain. Health is within your reach. Don't wait until you have an unhealthy condition. Commit to and follow Your Health Program. Enjoy good health now by using the programs offered in this book.

We are here to experience life and grow. We don't know when we are leaving this beautiful planet. Treasure your health while you are here and enjoy every moment of your life. It is your right as a human being. Respect others' rights also, for we are all here sharing the human experience together, and are learning from each other.

EAT HEALTHY. BE HEALTHY.

To your health! Namaste, Jane Falke

PART III
Recipes for Healthful Living

Recipes for Healthful Living

The suggested menu plan in The Maintenance Program follows the 75/25 rule for healthy eating. The recipes below use whole, natural, plant-based foods. You can adapt your favorite recipes easily to use these foods as I have done with several of them. Feel free to add your favorite vegetables, herbs, and spices as substitutes for others, and to make the recipes your own.

Some packaged foods are okay to use in your recipes if they are whole foods without added chemicals. Look at the ingredients list before you decide to buy. For instance, you can use tomatoes or tomato sauce if it comes in a bottle or a BPA-free can (BPA, or bisphenol A, is a toxin used to line the insides of cans), and if the ingredients are only tomatoes and fresh herbs. I often use canned beans in my recipes when I do not have time to cook them from scratch. I buy Eden Organics brand because they come in BPA-free cans. Read the labels or email the manufacturer before buying canned products to be sure they come in BPA-free cans. Or use products that come in cartons or glass jars or bottles.

Preparing these recipes at home ensures that you are eating the highest quality food available. You control what you eat and you know the quality of your meal.

If you do a little research on your local restaurants, you may find several items on their menus that fit the guidelines of The Maintenance Program. For instance, a fast-food restaurant in my city called Chipotle Grill offers fresh, low-fat, mostly organic ingredients for their tacos, burritos, and bowls. They also offer two types of beans – black and pinto – and brown and white rice. Their food is delicious, too.

Enjoy your health and energy with these recipes. You can find even more recipes on my website, www. janefalke.com/recipes. You can also follow my blog,

Eat Healthy. Be Healthy at Any Age.

sign up for my monthly newsletter, or sign up for my FREE guide called Discover What Food Labels Don't Tell You That Is Keeping You Fat, Sick, and Sluggish.

The Mini-Cleanse Recipes

Alkaline Power
6 celery stalks
1 cucumber, chopped
¼ bunch parsley
2 large collard greens

Cucumber Salad in a Glass
2 large cucumbers
½ tsp. salt
¼ lemon
1 inch fresh ginger
4 mint leaves

A Glass of Salad
8 romaine lettuce leaves
2 carrots
1 green onion
½ cucumber
½ red pepper
2 celery stalks
1 tomato
2 radishes
¼ lemon, peeled

Immune Booster
2 carrots
6 celery stalks
1 cucumber
3 handfuls spinach
¼ bunch parsley
¼ beet
2 tomatoes
½ lemon, peeled
1 inch fresh ginger root
1 green onion

Eat Healthy. Be Healthy at Any Age.

1 small garlic clove
dash cayenne pepper

Mineral Power
6 celery stalks
2 cucumbers
½ lemon, peeled

The Energizer
6 celery stalks
1 green apple
2 large handfuls spinach
3 kale leaves
¼ bunch parsley
1 inch fresh ginger root

Liver Cleanse
3 large carrots
4 large handfuls spinach
2 celery stalks
½ inch fresh turmeric root

The recipes below are adapted from *The Juice Lady's Guide to Juicing for Health* by Cherie Calbom, MS.

Popeye Power
2 handfuls spinach
¼ bunch parsley
3 carrots with skins
2 stalks celery
½ beet with skin

Triple C
½ head green cabbage
2 carrots
5 stalks celery

The recipe below is adapted from www. vegetablejuicerecipes.org

V8 Tomato Juice
3 tomatoes
3 carrots
½ small beet
3 stalks of celery
1 large handful spinach
1 red pepper
3 large kale leaves

The recipe below is adapted from www.myjuicecleanse. com

Green Power Juice
1 green apple
3 handfuls spinach
8 kale leaves
3 carrots
½ inch fresh ginger

The recipe below came from www.jointhereboot.com

Mean Green Juice
6 kale leaves
1 cucumber
4 celery stalks
2 green apples
½ lemon
1 inch fresh ginger

Eat Healthy. Be Healthy at Any Age.

The Cleansing Program Recipes

Fresh Almond Milk – makes 4 cups

Almond milk is so easy to make and better for you than pasteurized versions in cartons. If you use packaged almond milk, use the unsweetened kind.

>1 cup almonds, raw and organic (soaked)
>4 cups water, filtered

Soak the almonds about eight hours in filtered water in a glass jar. Using a draining screen, rinse a few times during the soak. Drain well before blending. Place the water and soaked almonds in a blender and blend for at least 1 minute. If you don't have a high-speed blender, blend longer. Strain the milk to remove the excess nut fiber. Throw away the fiber. Put the milk in a jar and refrigerate. It will keep for four to five days.

Flavored Almond Milk

>10-12 oz. Fresh Almond Milk
>½ tsp. vanilla
>1 package stevia powder

Stir together or blend.

Hemp Milk – makes 1 cup

This milk is high in protein and omega 3 fats. It's so easy to make. No soaking is necessary. Use instead of almond milk.

>2 tbsp. hemp seeds
>1 cup water

Blend together until smooth.

Smoothie Recipes

The Energy Drink – makes 3 cups

   8 oz. almond milk, hemp milk or water
   ½ cucumber, chopped
   ½ avocado, pitted and skinned
   5 large leaves kale
   3 stems of fresh mint or 3 drops of mint extract
   1 tbsp. flax, or chia seeds
   ½ lemon, juiced
   ½ tsp. sea salt
   1 package stevia powder
   dash cayenne pepper

Blend all ingredients until smooth.

The Energy Drink, Too – makes 3 cups

   8 oz. almond milk, hemp milk or water
   ½ cucumber, chopped
   1 stalk celery, chopped
   1 inch fresh ginger root, chopped
   ½ avocado, pitted and skinned
   1 large handful spinach
   1 tbsp. flax, or chia seeds
   ½ lemon, juiced
   ½ tsp. sea salt
   dash cayenne pepper

Blend all ingredients until smooth.

Green Coconut Smoothie – makes 3 cups

This is a sweeter version than the smoothies above.

   1 Thai coconut (meat), or use ½ package
   organic creamed coconut

Eat Healthy. Be Healthy at Any Age.

1 cup coconut water from the Thai coconut, or
  purified water with creamed coconut
½ cucumber, chopped
1 large handful spinach
1 tbsp. flax, chia, or hemp seeds
½ tsp. sea salt

Blend all ingredients until smooth.

Coconut Almond Milkshake – makes 3 cups

This recipe came from www.wholebodycleansing.net

1 Thai coconut (meat and water), or ½ package
  organic creamed coconut plus 1 cup purified
  water
1 cup almond milk
½ tsp. vanilla
1 package stevia powder

Blend ingredients until smooth. The shake will thicken
in the refrigerator.

If you need something to chew, try the following recipes.
Chew into a liquid before swallowing.

Guacamole – makes ¾ to 1 cup

1 avocado, pitted and skinned
½ tsp. sea salt
½ lemon, juiced

Smash the avocado in a bowl. Add the other ingredients.
Mix thoroughly.

Alkaline Salad – makes 1 ½ cups

½ cucumber, peeled, seeded, and diced
½ tomato, cored and diced
½ avocado, pitted, skinned, and diced

¼ tsp. sea salt
olive oil
dash cayenne pepper

Mix the cucumber, tomato, and avocado in a bowl. Top with the olive oil, salt, and cayenne pepper.

Luncheon Salad – makes 1 serving

Use any kind of dark leafy greens and add four or five different raw vegetables such as radishes, sprouts, tomatoes, cucumbers, avocados, celery, shredded zucchini, carrots or red cabbage.

For the Dressing:

2 tbsp. olive oil
1 tbsp. lemon juice
2 tsp. Bragg® Liquid Aminos™
Dash cayenne pepper

In a small bowl mix together all dressing ingredients. Sprinkle over salad and mix well. Don't forget to chew your salad into a liquid before swallowing.

Soup Recipes

The recipes below came from *Back to the House of Health,* by Shelley Young. I simplified some recipes for easy preparation.

Cucumber Avocado Soup – makes 1 serving

1 cucumber, chopped
1 avocado, pitted and skinned
¼ clove garlic, chopped
1 tsp. fresh lemon, juiced
sea salt to taste

Blend all ingredients until creamy.

Eat Healthy. Be Healthy at Any Age.

Celery Cauliflower Soup – makes 4 cups

¼ onion, peeled and chopped
¼ head of celery, trimmed and chopped
¼ head cauliflower, cored and chopped
2 cups vegetable broth
½ tsp. sea salt
1 cup almond milk
seasoning of your choice

Place all the ingredients except almond milk in a pot and simmer for 5 minutes. Add the almond milk and mix well. Puree until smooth. Drizzle with olive oil and a dash of cayenne pepper or seasoning of your choice.

No Tortilla Soup – makes 4 cups

This recipe came from Cheri Freeman and appeared in *Back to the House of Health 2* by Shelley Redford Young.

3 cups vegetable broth
3 large roma tomatoes, chopped
1 garlic clove, chopped
2 jalapeno peppers, seeded and chopped
¼ cup cilantro, chopped
¼ onion, chopped
1 stalk celery, chopped
sea salt
1 avocado, diced

Place all the ingredients except the avocado in a pot. Simmer on medium-low heat for 2 minutes. Puree until smooth. Top with avocado.

The following soup recipes I made-up while on the cleanse. Hope you enjoy them!

Creamy Broccoli Soup – makes 4 cups

½ medium onion, chopped
1 ½ cups vegetable broth
1 large head broccoli, florets and stems,
    chopped
sea salt
½ cup almond milk
dash cayenne pepper

Put everything in a pot except the almond milk and the cayenne. Bring to a boil. Cover and simmer on medium-low heat for 3 to 4 minutes. Add the almond milk and the cayenne pepper. Blend until smooth. Add more vegetable broth for a thinner consistency.

Rich Tomato Soup – makes 4 cups

1 pint cherry tomatoes
4 sun-dried tomatoes – not bottled – soaked in
    water for 10 minutes
1 cup warm purified water
1 clove garlic, chopped
½ tsp. each dried basil, oregano, and thyme
sea salt

Blend everything until thick and smooth. Add more water for a thinner consistency. Serve with a drizzle of olive oil and a dash of cayenne pepper.

Eat Healthy. Be Healthy at Any Age.

The Maintenance Program Recipes

Beverages

(Use any of the beverages in The Cleansing Program.)

Chai Coconut Tea – makes 1 cup

1 Yerba Maté Chai tea bag
8 oz. hot water
Coconut Milk (recipe below) or almond milk
stevia to taste

Put the ingredients in a cup and enjoy.

Coconut Milk – makes 4 cups

This is an option to fresh Thai coconut meat and its water.

1 package creamed coconut
4 cups water

Blend the ingredients for 2 minutes until smooth and strain. Put it in a glass bottle and refrigerate. Shake before using.

Lemon-Aid – makes 2 servings

Recipe from The Food Matters Cookbook by Mark Bittman

1 quart water
2 lemons, juiced
pinch of sea salt
1 inch fresh ginger root, peeled and pressed in
   a garlic press
stevia to taste

Mix in a pitcher and enjoy.

138

Spiced Grapefruit Cooler – makes 2 servings

Recipe from *The Food Matters Cookbook* by Mark Bittman

  3 yellow grapefruits, peeled, cored, and seeded
  ½ inch ginger root, peeled
  1 tsp. cinnamon
  1 tsp. vanilla extract
  6 ice cubes
  ¾ cup water
  stevia to taste

Blend on high until smooth.

Lemon Tea – makes 1 large cup

  10 oz. hot water
  ½ lemon, juiced
  stevia

Put the ingredients in a cup and enjoy.

Tomato Juice – makes 3 cups

  8 medium tomatoes
  1/2 cup water
  2 tbsp. onion, coarsely chopped
  2 celery stalks
  3 stems parsley
  1 tsp. salt
  1/4 tsp. paprika

Blend, strain, and chill.

Eat Healthy. Be Healthy at Any Age.

Breakfast Foods

- Quinoa flakes and cream of buckwheat are available at most health food stores. Add almond milk, cinnamon, and chopped or sliced almonds for a tasty and hearty breakfast.
- All of the smoothies in The Cleansing Program are great for breakfast.
- Fruit contains many alkaline minerals and a natural sugar called fructose. Fruit metabolizes as acids because of the sugar content, so it can deplete alkaline minerals. But sugar is sugar, and as you may recall, sugar can cause addictions and cravings. Be careful about what kinds of fruits you eat and how much. Fruits with low sugar content such as berries, apples, and pears are acceptable on occasion when you are balanced.

Berry Smoothie – makes 3 cups

Use this recipe occasionally when you are balanced.

½ cup fresh or frozen strawberries or
    blueberries
10 oz. almond milk
1 tbsp. chia, hemp, or flax seeds
4 drops liquid stevia or coconut crystals

Blend all the ingredients on high for 1 minute.

Breakfast Quinoa with Berries and Almonds

Adapted from *The Homesteader's Kitchen* by Robin Burnside.

1 ½ cups water
½ tsp. sea salt

1 cup quinoa, rinsed and drained
1 cup berries, any kind
¼ cup almonds, chopped or sliced
¼ cup almond milk

Boil the water in a saucepan and add the salt and quinoa. Cover and cook on low for 15 minutes. Let it sit for 5 minutes. Serve with berries, almonds, and almond milk.

Broccoli, Tomato, and Avocado – makes 2 servings

A lettuce-free meal that is easy to prepare.

2 cups broccoli florets
1 tomato, diced
1 avocado, diced
1 tsp. olive oil
1 tbsp. sliced almonds or seeds of choice
2 dashes sea salt and sprinkle with Spice
    Hunter's The Zip® or cayenne pepper

Blanch the broccoli in hot water for 2 to 3 minutes. Drain and rinse it in cold water. Place in a bowl the broccoli, tomato, then the avocado. Drizzle with olive oil. Top with almonds, salt, and Spice Hunter's The Zip®.

Creamy Buckwheat Cereal with Cinnamon, Vanilla, and Almonds

½ cup Bob's Red Mill Creamy Buckwheat
    Cereal™
1 ¼ cups water
¼ to ½ tsp. ground cinnamon
½ tsp. vanilla extract
almond milk
coconut crystals
almonds, chopped or slivered

Follow the package directions for making the cereal. Stir in the cinnamon and vanilla. Add the almond milk. Sprinkle with the coconut crystals and top with the almonds.

French Toast with Coconut Syrup – makes 2 servings

Coconut Syrup:

½ cup coconut water
½ package creamed coconut plus ½ cup water
1 tsp. vanilla
4 drops liquid stevia

French Toast:

1 cup Rich Almond Milk (see recipe below)
½ tsp. vanilla extract
dash or 2 of cinnamon
½ package stevia powder
1 ½ tsp. coconut oil
6 slices Manna brand bread (whole grain,
    millet or sun seed)

Blend all the ingredients for the Coconut Syrup until smooth. Add more water if necessary. Blend all the ingredients for the French Toast, except the bread, and mix thoroughly. Pour into a shallow dish, add the bread, and soak it for 5 minutes on each side. Heat a skillet. Add the coconut oil. Add the bread and cook on medium-low heat until slightly brown on both sides. Serve with the Coconut Syrup.

Rich Almond Milk:

Make the Fresh Almond Milk recipe only use 2 cups of water instead of 4 cups.

Granola – makes 5 cups

From www.phmiracleliving.com by Michael Steadman

This recipe is great as a snack or as a cereal with Fresh Almond Milk.

1 cup almonds, soaked overnight
½ cup pecans, soaked 1 hour
½ cup walnuts, soaked 1 hour
½ cup macadamia nuts
½ cup pine nuts
1 cup unsweetened dried coconut flakes
½ cup mesquite powder, optional
¼ cup ground cinnamon
1 tsp. sea salt
1 tbsp. stevia powder

In a food processor, pulse the soaked nuts until coarsely ground. Place them in a mixing bowl, add the remaining ingredients, and mix well. Place them on a Teflex dehydrator sheet and dehydrate at 110 degrees for 36 hours, or until crisp. Or bake in the oven at the lowest temperature for about 3 hours until crisp.

Millet Porridge – makes 2 servings

Adapted recipe from *The Food Matters Cookbook* by Mark Bittman

½ cup millet
1/8 tsp. sea salt
½ tsp. cinnamon
¼ tsp. cardamom powder
almond milk
stevia or coconut crystals
½ cup berries, sliced
¼ cup almonds, chopped

Rinse and drain the millet. Put it in a pot with 1 ¼ cups water and the cinnamon and cardamom. Bring it to a simmer, cover, and cook on low until the water is absorbed, about 15 minutes. Add almond milk, sweetener, berries, and chopped almonds.

Pumpkin Smoothie – makes 3 cups

Adapted from *Food for Life* by Neil Barnard, recipe by Mary Ohno, www.pcrm.org

½ pumpkin puree, no sugar (from carton)
1 cup almond milk
1 cup ice
1 tsp. vanilla extract
1 tsp. pumpkin pie spice
stevia to taste

Blend all the ingredients until smooth.

Quinoa with Avocado, Tomatoes, and Almonds – makes 2 servings

½ cup quinoa, rinsed
1 ½ cups water
½ tsp. sea salt
olive oil
½ avocado
½ tomato
1/8 cup almonds, sliced or chopped

Bring the water to a boil. Add the quinoa, lower the heat, and simmer covered for 15 minutes. Let stand for 5 minutes. Scoop ¾ cup into a bowl and drizzle with oil. Top with the avocado, tomato, and almonds. You can also add sprouts, a dash of cayenne, or sprinkle on Spice Hunter's The Zip®.

Scrambled Tofu with Spinach – makes 2 servings

Inspired by *Simple Suppers* from the Moosewood collection of recipe books.

1 tbsp. coconut oil
1/3 cup onions, finely chopped
6 oz. firm sprouted tofu, crumbled
1 tbsp. Bragg® Liquid Aminos™
½ tsp. garlic granules
½ tsp. turmeric
¼ tsp. cumin, ground
2 cups spinach, chopped

Heat the oil in a non-stick skillet. Add the onions and cook over medium heat, stirring often, for 1 minute. Add the spinach, cover, and steam for 1 minute. Use a fork to mash the tofu with the Bragg's on a flat plate. Add the tofu, garlic, turmeric, and cumin, and cook stirring gently for 1 minute. You can eat as is or wrap in a sprouted whole wheat tortilla for a delicious breakfast burrito.

Salads and Soups

- Soups and salads are always a hit for lunch or dinner. Baby spinach, mixed greens, and dark, leafy lettuces are best for salads. Be sure to add many alkaline vegetables like avocado, tomato, sprouts, cabbage, jicama, green or red onions, cucumber, celery, radishes, bell peppers, and such. For taste and variety, try salsa, vegan pesto, or any of the dressings in the recipe section.
- In The Maintenance Program, you will not have to puree your soups as you did in The Cleansing Program. Prepare them as usual or add any alkaline vegetables you like, but instead of

roughly chopping them, dice or chop them in ways that provide a good presentation, making your soup appealing.

- If you have a Vitamix blender, it likely came with a recipe book. Go through it and pick out the recipes that attract you. They adapt easily for an alkaline plant meal. For instance, you can use almond milk instead of cow's milk or cream, omit mushrooms and add another vegetable instead, use vegetable broth instead of chicken broth, or use lemon juice instead of vinegar.
- One night a week can be Soup and Salad Night. Pick from the recipes below and you will have a healthy and complete alkaline meal.

Salads

Asian Slaw with Wasabi Dressing – makes 2 servings

Dressing:

2 tbsp. Bragg® Liquid Aminos™
2 tbsp. lemon juice
1 clove garlic, minced
1 tbsp. ginger, peeled and minced
1 tsp. wasabi powder
1 tbsp. sesame oil, toasted

Whisk all the Dressing ingredients together in a small bowl.

Slaw:

2 cups Napa or Savoy cabbage, finely sliced
2 cups bok choy, leaves cut in half lengthwise
and thinly sliced crosswise

1 cup carrots, grated
¼ red onion, thinly sliced

Put the Slaw ingredients in a large bowl. Add the Dressing and toss well. Let it marinate in the refrigerator for 15 minutes.

Asparagus Salad with Mustard Dressing – makes 4 servings

Dressing:

½ small shallot, chopped
½ garlic clove, chopped
1/8 cup lemon juice
1 tsp. dried mustard
¼ tsp. sea salt
¼ cup olive oil

Place all the ingredients in a mini-blender and combine thoroughly.

Salad:

½ pound fresh asparagus, ends broken off,
    stalks cut diagonally into 1 inch pieces
2 celery stalks, cut into ¼ inch pieces
1 small carrot, shredded
1/8 cup fresh Italian parsley, finely chopped
1/8 cup fresh cilantro, finely chopped
1 roma tomato, seeded and diced

Blanch the asparagus in hot water for 2 minutes. Toss the Salad ingredients and Dressing in a bowl. Refrigerate for 15 minutes.

Eat Healthy. Be Healthy at Any Age.

Caesar Salad – makes 2 servings (and extra dressing)

Dressing:

1 small garlic clove, chopped
1/3 cup olive oil
1 tsp. dried mustard
1 ½ tsp. vegan Worcestershire sauce
¼ cup cashews, soaked for 15 minutes
1 ½ - 2 tbsp. fresh lemon juice
¼ tsp. salt

Blend all the Dressing ingredients for 1 minute.

Salad:

½ head romaine lettuce, washed, dried, and
    broken into bite-sized pieces
8 cherry tomatoes cut in half
1/8 cup chopped walnuts

Place the lettuce in a bowl. Toss it with some of the Dressing and top with tomatoes and walnuts.

Chopped Salad with Lemongrette Dressing – makes 2 servings (and extra dressing)

Dressing:

½ shallot, chopped
½ garlic clove, chopped
1 ½ tsp. dried mustard
5 drops liquid stevia
½ tsp. salt
¼ cup lemon juice
½ cup olive oil

Process the shallots and garlic in a food processor until minced. Add the mustard, stevia, salt, and lemon juice, and combine thoroughly. While the machine is running, slowly add the oil until smooth.

148

Salad:

1 cup jicama, peeled and cut into ½ inch cubes
½ cucumber, peeled, seeded and cut into ½
   inch cubes
½ red pepper, cut into ½ inch pieces
¼ cup red onions, chopped
½ head romaine lettuce, shredded
6 radishes, chopped

Put the Salad ingredients in a bowl. Add some Dressing and toss well.

Cucumber Salad – makes 2 servings

2 cucumbers, peeled and thinly sliced
1 tsp. sea salt
1 tbsp. lime juice
1 tsp. ginger, minced
1 tbsp. toasted sesame oil
2 drops liquid stevia
1 tbsp. mint, cut in thin strands
sesame seeds

Place the cucumbers in a strainer over a bowl and toss them with salt. Allow them to sit for a half hour, squeezing the liquid out occasionally. In a bowl, whisk the lime juice, ginger, oil, and stevia. Toss the dressing with the cucumbers and mint. Sprinkle with the sesame seeds.

Garden Wrap with Sweet Korean Dipping Sauce
– makes 2 wraps

Sauce:

3 tbsp. Bragg® Liquid Aminos™
3 tbsp. lemon juice
4 drops liquid stevia

Eat Healthy. Be Healthy at Any Age.

1 garlic clove, pressed
1 inch ginger root, pressed
3 tbsp. toasted sesame oil

Mix all the ingredients in a small bowl.

Wrap:

2 large collard or Swiss chard leaves
½ avocado, sliced
¼ cucumber, peeled, seeded, thinly sliced
½ carrot, shredded
½ zucchini, shredded
¼ red pepper, thinly sliced

Cut off the end of the chard stem. Lay the leaf on a cutting board with the back facing up. Horizontally slice off the thickest part of the stem near the bottom to flatten. Layer all ingredients on the back of the leaf. Roll them up burrito style, tucking in the ends. Slice the rolls into two pieces. Dip in Sauce.

Home-Style Carrot Salad – makes 2 servings

Adapted from *The Raw Gourmet*, by Nomi Shannon.

4 medium carrots, finely grated
1 tsp. lemon peel, grated
1 tbsp. lemon juice
1 tsp. olive oil
4 drops liquid stevia

Put the grated carrots in a bowl. Grate the lemon peel before juicing the lemon. In a small bowl, mix the rest of the ingredients. Add them to the carrots and mix thoroughly. Let it marinate in the refrigerator for an hour. Serve on a lettuce leaf.

Kale Slaw – makes 2 servings

Dressing:

> 2 tbsp. olive oil
> 1 tbsp. lemon juice
> 2 drops liquid stevia
> 1 small garlic clove, crushed
> 1 tsp. onion powder
> ¼ tsp. dried mustard
> dash cayenne pepper

Combine all the ingredients in a glass jar. Cover and shake to blend.

Salad:

> ½ bunch kale, stems removed, cut into thin ribbons
> ¼ tsp. sea salt
> ¼ head cabbage, shredded
> 1 roma tomato, seeded and diced
> 1/8 small red onion, finely julienned

In a large bowl, massage the kale with the salt for a couple of minutes to soften. Add the rest of ingredients and the Dressing, and toss well.

Mixed Greens with Lemongrette Dressing – makes 2 servings (and extra dressing)

Dressing:½ shallot, chopped

> ½ garlic clove, chopped
> 1 ½ tsp. dried mustard
> 5 drops liquid stevia
> ½ tsp. salt
> ¼ cup lemon juice
> ½ cup olive oil

Eat Healthy. Be Healthy at Any Age.

Process the shallots and garlic in a food processor until minced. Add the mustard, stevia, salt, and lemon juice, and combine thoroughly. While the machine is running, slowly add the oil until smooth.

Salad:

2 large handfuls mixed greens
1/8 red onion, thinly sliced
½ apple, chopped
¼ cup slivered almonds

Put the Salad ingredients in a bowl and toss with some of the Dressing.

Sweet and Spicy Kale Salad – makes 2 servings

Salad:

1 bunch of kale
¼ onion, diced
¼ tsp. salt
8 cherry tomatoes, halved
½ avocado, diced

Cut off the center rib from the kale and chop roughly. Place it in a large bowl with the onions and salt. Mix it well with your hands to soften the kale.

Dressing:

1/8 cup olive oil
1 ½ tbsp. lemon juice
5 drops liquid stevia
1 ½ tbsp. raw almond butter
1 tbsp. Bragg® Liquid Aminos™
2 dashes cayenne pepper

Mix the Dressing ingredients in a small bowl and pour it on top of the Salad. Massage all the ingredients well

152

with your hands. Let it marinate in the refrigerator for 30 minutes. Serve topped with tomatoes and avocados.

Spinach Salad – makes 2 servings

Salad:

6 oz. baby spinach, washed
1 large roma tomato cut in chunks
¼ red onion, thinly sliced
1 small cucumber, peeled, cut in half
    lengthwise, seeded, and thinly sliced
½ red bell pepper, thinly sliced

Put the Salad ingredients in a bowl.

Dressing:

3 tbsp. lemon juice
¼ cup olive oil
1 tbsp. Bragg® Liquid Aminos™
¼ tsp. oregano, dried
2 drops liquid stevia

Whisk the Dressing ingredients in a small bowl, add them to the Salad, and toss.

Three Bean Salad – makes 4 servings

½ pound fresh green beans, cut into 1 inch
    pieces
1 can (15 oz.) kidney beans, rinsed and
    drained
1 can (15 oz.) garbanzo beans, rinsed and
    drained
½ small red pepper, chopped
¼ small onion, chopped
2 tbsp. olive oil
½ fresh lemon, juiced

¼ tsp. dried oregano, crushed
4 drops liquid stevia
½ tsp. sea salt

Lightly steam the green beans for 3 minutes. Drain and rinse them under cold water. Place all the ingredients in a bowl and mix well. Refrigerate for 30 minutes to blend the flavors.

Tostada Salad – makes two 8 inch tostadas

2 sprouted whole wheat tortillas
½ cup refried beans
½ cup cooked brown rice, quinoa, or millet
2 handfuls sprouts or mixed lettuce
Guacamole
Salsa

Guacamole:

1 avocado, mashed
¼ tsp. sea salt
1 tsp. lime or lemon juice

Mix everything in a small bowl.

Salsa:

1 tomato, chopped
½ jalapeno pepper, seeds removed and chopped
2 tbsp. onion, chopped
1 garlic clove, chopped
1 tsp. lime or lemon juice
1 tsp. cilantro, chopped
¼ tsp. sea salt
1-2 dashes cayenne pepper

Lightly blend the Salsa ingredients in a mini-blender for 10 to 15 seconds. Warm the tortillas, put them on a plate, and spread them with the beans. Add the grains, sprouts or lettuce, avocado, and salsa. Fold in half or roll into a wrap.

Extra Dressings

Herb Dressing To Go – makes 1 cup

This dressing is great for taking with you. When you use dried herbs, no refrigeration is required. Add fresh lemon or lime juice when you're ready to use it. It will keep for a month without refrigeration. When you use fresh herbs, refrigerate. Keeps 10 days.

¾ cup olive oil
2 tsp. dry mustard
½ tsp. granulated garlic
1 tsp. sea salt
½ tsp. dry tarragon
½ tsp. dry thyme
2 tsp. The Spice Hunter Deliciously Dill™
   seasoning
dash cayenne pepper

Place the ingredients in a glass jar. Cover and shake up to mix.

Ranch Dressing

¼ cup raw cashews, soaked for 15 minutes and
   drained
¼ cup water
1 ½ tsp. lemon juice
¼ tsp. garlic granules
¼ tsp. sea salt
1 ½ tsp. The Spice Hunter Deliciously Dill™
   seasoning

Blend all the ingredients until creamy. Add water to thin.

Soups and Stews

Gazpacho Soup – makes 4 cups

This is an easy and fast recipe made in the blender.

  3 cups of vegetable broth
  2 large tomatoes, chopped
  1 cucumber
  ½ red pepper, seeded
  1 small jalapeno pepper, seeded
  1 celery stalk, chopped
  ½ lemon or lime juiced
  ½ tsp. ground cumin
  1 garlic clove, chopped
  1 tsp. sea salt
  ½ avocado, diced

Blend the ingredients, except the avocado, on medium power until chunky or high power until smooth. Chill in the refrigerator for 20 minutes. Serve topped with avocado.

Moroccan Vegetable Stew – makes 2 servings

Adapted from Martha Stewart's *Everyday Food: Great Food Fast.*

  ½ onion, cut in quarters and thinly sliced
  ¾ tsp. each ground turmeric, ground
    cinnamon, chili powder, and sea salt
  1 tbsp. fresh ginger, minced
  3 carrots, peeled and cut diagonally into ½
    inch thick slices
  3 large tomatoes, diced in 3/4 inch pieces
  1 cup vegetable broth
  1 zucchini, cut in half lengthwise, then
    diagonally in ½ inch slices

Heat a large pot. Add 1 tablespoon vegetable broth and sauté the onions for about 3 minutes. Add the turmeric, cinnamon, chili powder, salt, and ginger. Mix thoroughly into the onions and cook for a few minutes to blend the flavors. Add the carrots, tomatoes, and broth. Stir gently. Bring to a simmer, cover, and cook for 10 minutes. Add the zucchini and cook until crispy tender, about 3 to 4 minutes. Serve as is or over cooked quinoa, millet, or brown rice.

Navy Bean Soup – makes 4 servings

    2 cans navy beans, drained and rinsed
    3 cups vegetable broth
    ½ onion, chopped
    1 garlic clove, minced
    1 celery stalk, diced
    1 cup carrots, peeled and chopped
    1 cup kale, stemmed and chopped
    ½ tsp. thyme
    ½ tsp. sage
    ½ tsp. salt

Place all the ingredients in a large pot. Bring to a boil. Turn the heat to low. Cover and simmer for 10 to 15 minutes until carrots are cooked.

Tortilla Soup – makes 4 servings

This recipe was in The Cleansing Program as No Tortilla Soup; this is a heartier version. You can make the tortillas and tofu ahead of time. Adapted from Cheri Freeman's recipe in *Back to the House of Health 2* by Shelley Redford Young.

Tortillas:

    2 sprouted whole wheat tortillas
    coconut oil
    sea salt

Eat Healthy. Be Healthy at Any Age.

Heat the oven to 350 degrees. Brush the tortillas on both sides with the coconut oil and salt them lightly. Stack them on top of one another and cut into thirds, then cut them in thin strips. Spread the strips out on a baking sheet and bake for about 8 to 10 minutes until crispy. Let cool.

Tofu:

    8-10 oz. tofu, diced into 1 inch cubes
    2 tbsp. Bragg® Liquid Aminos™
    1 garlic clove, minced
    ¼ tsp. crushed red chili peppers

While the tortillas are crisping in the oven, marinate the tofu in the Bragg's, garlic, and chili peppers, tossing every few minutes. Heat a skillet on medium high, add the tofu, and lightly brown, turning over occasionally.

Soup:

    4 cups vegetable broth
    2 cups fresh pureed roma tomatoes or store-bought diced or strained tomatoes
    2 tbsp. garlic, minced
    ½ cup cilantro, finely chopped
    ½ onion, finely chopped
    ½ tsp. sea salt
    1 zucchini, diced
    ¼ to ½ cup fresh salsa, medium heat
    1 avocado, diced

Pour the broth and tomato puree in a saucepan and heat until simmering. Add the tofu, garlic, cilantro, onions, salt, zucchini, and salsa. Heat for 2 to 3 minutes. Serve topped with avocado and tortilla strips.

Main Meals

Brown Rice Bowl with Marinated Tofu and Vegetables – makes 2 servings

You can make the Marinated Tofu ahead of time and store it in the refrigerator. Use the leftover Marinated Tofu on top of your luncheon salads or eat as a snack.

Marinated Tofu:

3 tbsp. Bragg® Liquid Aminos™
1 clove garlic, minced
½ inch piece fresh ginger, peeled and minced
2 tsp. toasted sesame oil
¼ tsp. crushed red chili flakes
1 tsp. sesame seeds, white or black
10 oz. tofu, extra firm, cut in 1 inch cubes

Preheat the oven to 450 degrees. Place in a bowl and add the Bragg's, garlic, ginger, oil, chili, and seeds. Mix thoroughly. Put the cut-up tofu in the bowl and marinate for 15 minutes or more, turning often. Put the drained tofu on an oil-sprayed baking pan. Keep the leftover marinade to add to the Brown Rice Bowl. Bake the tofu for 10 minutes, turn it over and bake it for another 10 minutes.

Brown Rice Bowl:

1 ½ cups brown rice, cooked
1 cup carrots, peeled and cut diagonally into ¼ inch slices
1 cup broccoli florets
½ red pepper, seeded and diced

Cook the brown rice according to the package directions. Lightly steam the carrots, broccoli, and red peppers for about 3 minutes. Place the rice in two bowls and

Eat Healthy. Be Healthy at Any Age.

add the vegetables and some tofu cubes. Top with the leftover marinade and serve with extra Bragg's.

Udon Noodles with Steam-Fried Vegetables –
makes 4 servings

  8 oz. udon noodles
  3+ tbsp. vegetable broth
  2 garlic cloves, minced
  ¼ tsp. red pepper flakes
  1 medium head bok choy, cut into 1 x 2 inch pieces
  2 cups broccoli florets
  2 medium carrots, julienned
  ½ cup snap peas or Chinese pea pods cut
    diagonally in half
  3 tbsp. Bragg® Liquid Aminos™
  2 tbsp. sesame oil, toasted

Cook the noodles according to the package directions. Drain and rinse them with cold water. Heat a skillet on high and add 3 tablespoons broth. When simmering, add the garlic and red pepper flakes and stir-fry for 1 minute. Add the broccoli and carrots, and more broth if needed. Stir-fry the vegetables for 1 minute. Add the bok choy and pea pods. Stir-fry for 1 more minute. Cover and cook for 3 minutes. Add the cooked noodles, Bragg's, and sesame oil. Toss lightly and cook uncovered for 2 more minutes.

Marinated Skewered Vegetables over Brown Rice – makes 6 skewers

Marinade:

  3 tbsp. Bragg® Liquid Aminos™
  3 tbsp. lemon juice
  4 drops liquid stevia
  2 garlic cloves, pressed
  1 inch ginger root, pressed

3 tbsp. toasted sesame oil
¼ tsp. crushed red chili peppers

Mix all the ingredients in a bowl.

Vegetables:

¼ small eggplant, cut into 1 ½ inch cubes
¼ cauliflower, cut in 1 ½ inch florets and
 blanched
1 red pepper, cut in 1 ½ inch pieces
1 zucchini, halved lengthwise and cut into 1 ½
 inch pieces
½ red onion cut into wedges
1 ½ cups brown rice, cooked

Add Vegetables to the bowl with the Marinade. Toss, cover, and marinate for 30 minutes. Heat the oven to broil. Put the Vegetables on wooden skewers and broil for 10 minutes, turning often. Serve over cooked brown rice or quinoa and drizzle with the leftover marinade.

Pasta Primavera – makes 3 servings

½ package whole wheat or brown rice penne
 pasta
1 cup broccoli florets
1 zucchini, cut into half moons about ½ inch thick
½ red pepper, julienned
1 cup frozen peas or fresh snap peas, cut into 1
 inch pieces
1 tbsp. vegetable broth
1 garlic clove, minced
¼ tsp. dried oregano
¼ tsp. crushed red chili pepper, optional
olive oil for finishing

Boil salted water for the pasta. Add the vegetables except the peas. Simmer for 3 minutes. Scoop out

Eat Healthy. Be Healthy at Any Age.

the vegetables into a bowl and set them aside. Cook the pasta in the same boiling water according to the package directions. Reserve ½ cup of pasta water. Rinse and drain. Heat a sauté pan on medium. Add the vegetable broth, garlic, chili, and oregano. Sauté for 1 minute. Add the steamed vegetables, pasta water, pasta, and peas. Mix well. Serve in bowls and drizzle with olive oil.

Pasta with Roasted Zucchini, Tomatoes, and Onions – makes 3 servings

Adapted from *Martha Stewart's Everyday Food: Great Food Fast.*

> 2 medium zucchinis, cut in half lengthwise, then cut crosswise into 1 inch pieces
> ½ large onion, halved crosswise and cut into ½ inch wedges
> 1 pint cherry tomatoes
> ½ tsp. sea salt
> 1/8 cup avocado oil
> ½ pound dried whole wheat or brown rice penne, ribbon, or fusilli pasta
> ½ cup crushed tomatoes

Heat the oven to 450 degrees. Put the zucchini, onions, and tomatoes in a roasting pan. Add the salt and oil and toss well to coat. Place these in the oven and roast until tender, about 20 minutes, tossing the vegetables about half way through. Meanwhile, cook the pasta in boiling salted water according to the package instructions. Reserve ½ cup of the pasta water, drain the pasta, and return it to the pot. Add the roasted vegetables, pasta water, and crushed tomatoes. Toss well and serve.

Recipes for Healthful Living

Sesame Tofu with Spinach – makes 2 servings

Adapted from *Simple Suppers* from the Moosewood collection of recipe books.

8 oz. firm tofu cut in 1 inch cubes
¼ cup sesame seeds
1 tbsp. sesame oil, toasted
1 tbsp. Bragg® Liquid Aminos™
a few drops of hot pepper sauce or a dash of
    cayenne pepper
1 tsp. coconut oil
1 large garlic clove, minced
6 oz. fresh baby spinach, rinsed but not dried
sea salt

Spread the sesame seeds on a plate and press all the surfaces of the tofu into the seeds to coat them evenly. Heat the sesame oil in a large skillet on medium heat, add the tofu in a single layer, and cook for 5 minutes. Turn the tofu over and cook for 5 more minutes. Add the Bragg's and hot pepper sauce. Turn the tofu over and cook for 1 minute. Remove the tofu to a plate. To the pan add the coconut oil and garlic and sauté for 30 seconds. Add the wet spinach and cook for 1 minute, stirring constantly. Sprinkle with salt. Place the spinach on plates and top with the tofu.

Stuffed Vegetables with Marinara Sauce – makes 2 servings

You can substitute eggplant or delicate squash for the bell peppers.

2 large red, yellow, or orange bell peppers,
    topped, seeded, and cored
1 tbsp. coconut oil
½ small onion, chopped
1 garlic clove, minced

163

¼ tsp. crushed red chili peppers
1 medium zucchini, chopped
1 roma tomato, seeded and chopped
1 tbsp. fresh oregano, chopped
1 tsp. sea salt
½ cup brown rice or quinoa, cooked
1 jar of prepared marinara sauce

Sprinkle the insides of the peppers with salt and replace the tops. (If using eggplant, scoop the middle section out, leaving about 1 inch of seed-free skin. Sprinkle with salt to leach the bitter liquid and dab dry with a paper towel before stuffing. If using squash, scoop the seeds out and sprinkle with salt.) Bake the salted vegetables at 400 degrees for 10 minutes.

Heat the oil over medium heat. Add the onions and sauté for 3 minutes. Add the garlic and red pepper flakes and sauté for 1 minute. Add the zucchini, tomatoes, oregano, and salt. Cover and cook for 5 minutes. In a bowl, combine the stuffing ingredients with the rice. Fill the peppers with the stuffing and bake for 12 minutes.

Tofu and Eggplant – makes 2 servings

Adapted from *Simple Suppers* from the Moosewood collection of recipe books

1 tbsp. avocado oil
2 garlic cloves, minced
½ red pepper, chopped
½ tsp. dried oregano
½ tsp. salt
1 cup vegetable broth
8 oz. firm tofu, cut into ¾ inch cubes
6 oz. eggplant, peeled and cut into 1 inch cubes
1 cup green beans, cut 1 inch pieces
1 cup roma tomatoes, diced

2 tbsp. fresh basil, chopped
sea salt

In a skillet over medium heat, sauté the oil and garlic for 30 seconds. Add the bell pepper, oregano, and salt. Cook for 3 minutes, stirring occasionally. Add the broth and tofu. Cook on high heat for 4 minutes to reduce the liquid. Add the eggplant, green beans, and tomatoes. Cook on medium heat for 5 minutes, stirring occasionally. Add the basil and salt. Toss and serve.

Vegetables in Parchment – makes 2 servings

2 pieces parchment paper about 16 x 16 inches
   each
2 large handfuls of baby spinach
1 carrot, julienned
½ zucchini, julienned
1 cup asparagus or green beans (about 6
   stalks) cut into 1 inch pieces
½ red bell pepper, julienned
½ tsp. salt
¼ cup vegetable broth

Heat the oven to 400 degrees. Place the parchment paper on a baking pan. Place one large handful of spinach in the center of the paper. Add ½ of the vegetables on top of the spinach and sprinkle with salt. Bring the two sides of the parchment paper together starting at the top, overlapping the folded edge several times as you go. Then fold one end several times to secure it. Pour ½ the vegetable broth into the open end of each pocket, then fold to secure it. Bake for about 20 minutes.

Healthy Snacks

* Raw, soaked nuts can be prepared overnight. Place the desired amount of nuts in a glass

container and cover with purified water. Refrigerate overnight. Rinse and drain the next morning. Store in the refrigerator and rinse daily, or dehydrate them for a crunchy texture.

- Raw vegetables such as cherry tomatoes, carrot sticks, celery sticks, jicama, radishes, and red peppers are good for increasing your intake of vegetables. Use a dipping sauce or Ranch Dressing (see salad recipes).
- Make Sprouted Whole Wheat Tortilla Chips ahead of time. Store them in the pantry. Dip them in salsa, hummus, or guacamole.
- Suzie's Spelt Puffed Cakes™, Savory Seed Crackers, or celery stalks with almond butter make crunchy treats. Spread raw almond butter, pâté, or smashed avocado on the cakes or crackers.
- Sprouted sunflower seeds or pumpkin seeds sprinkled with sea salt are good for an immediate snack. You can buy these at a natural food store or make them in your dehydrator.

Guacamole Dip – makes 2 cups

2 avocados, pitted and skin removed
2 roma tomatoes, seeded and chopped
¼ cup fresh cilantro, chopped
¼ small red onion, chopped
2 garlic cloves, minced
½ jalapeno pepper, minced
1 tbsp. lime juice
dash cayenne pepper
1 tsp. sea salt

In a bowl, mash the avocado with a fork. Add all the ingredients and mix well. Serve with dehydrated Savory Seed Crackers, Sprouted Whole Wheat Tortilla Chips, or raw veggies.

Healthy Trail Mix – makes 3 cups

½ cup sunflower seeds
¼ cup pumpkin seeds
¼ cup sesame seeds, white
½ cup almonds
¼ cup macadamia nuts, chopped
¼ cup Bragg® Liquid Aminos™
1 tsp. garlic granules
4 dashes cayenne pepper

Put the seeds and almonds in a sprouting jar. Rinse and drain at least 3 times. Fill the jar with purified water to cover. Add the Bragg's, garlic, and cayenne. Mix thoroughly. Cover and let soak for 6 hours or overnight. Drain and rinse. Spread on mesh dehydrator trays. Dehydrate at 110 degrees for 6 to 8 hours until crispy. Alternatively, bake in the oven at the lowest temperature for 3 hours or until crispy. Put in an airtight container. They will last for one month. Eat as a snack or sprinkle over salads.

Marinated Sunflower Seeds – makes 2 cups

1 ½ cups raw sunflower seeds
3 tbsp. Bragg® Liquid Aminos™
1 tsp. garlic granules

Soak the seeds in a sprouting jar for 4 hours or more. Rinse and drain a few times. Mix the Bragg's and garlic granules in a bowl. Add the seeds, mix well, and marinate for 15 to 30 minutes. To dehydrate: spread the seeds on a Teflex dehydrator sheet and dehydrate at 110 degrees for 8 to 10 hours until crispy. To bake: spread the seeds on a cookie sheet at the lowest temperature in the oven for 2 to 3 hours until crispy.

Eat Healthy. Be Healthy at Any Age.

Savory Seed Crackers – Dehydrate or Bake - makes about 50 crackers

Adapted from *Dr. Mercola's Total Health Program.*

1 cup sesame seeds, hulled
½ cup sunflower seeds
¼ cup golden flax seeds
1 tsp. garlic granules
1 tsp. Herbamare® Original
2 tsp. The Spice Hunter Deliciously Dill™
  seasoning
1 celery stalk, chopped
parchment paper

Soak the seeds together for 6 hours or overnight. Rinse and drain. In a food processor, place the garlic, Herbamare® Original, dill seasoning, and celery, and process until ground. Add the soaked seeds and process until well mixed and smooth.

Roll half the dough between two pieces of parchment paper (if baking) or between Teflex dehydrator sheets (if dehydrating). Roll with a rolling pin until ¼ inch thick. Carefully peel off the top sheet. Using a spatula, shape the dough into a square or rectangle, leveling out the edges. Score into cracker-sized pieces, 2 x 2 inches. Prepare the remaining dough as above.

To dehydrate, place Teflex sheet on dehydrator tray and dehydrate at 110 degrees for 12 hrs.

To bake, place the parchment paper on a cookie sheet. Bake at the lowest oven heat setting until crispy, about 4 hours. Let cool.

Break the crackers apart, put in an airtight jar, and store in the pantry for up to 2 months.

Spread smashed avocado or hummus on top, eat with salads, or crumble over soups and salads.

Walnut Pâté – makes 1 cup

1 cup walnuts, soaked 20 minutes, rinsed, and
  drained
1 small clove garlic
1 tbsp. onion, chopped
1 celery stalk, chopped
¼ cup parsley, stems removed and chopped
1 tbsp. fresh lemon juice
½ tsp. sea salt

In a food processor, finely chop the garlic, onions,
celery, and parsley. Add the walnuts, juice, and salt.
Blend until smooth.

Stuff cherry tomatoes, spread on crackers, or add as a
side to a salad.

Sprouted Whole Wheat Tortilla Chips – makes 4 servings

From www.phmiracleliving.com

¾ package sprouted whole wheat tortillas
coconut oil
sea salt

Brush or spray the tortillas on both sides with coconut
oil and sprinkle with sea salt. Stack the tortillas on top
of each other and cut up into pie-shaped pieces. Place
them on a baking sheets and toast at 375 degrees for
about ten minutes.

Dip these chips in salsa, hummus, or guacamole.

APPENDIX 1

The Glycemic Index

The glycemic index (GI) rates carbohydrate-containing foods according to their effect on your body's blood sugar. Low-fiber and processed foods raise blood sugar quickly and have a high GI rating – between 100 and 150. High-fiber foods and whole foods move more slowly through the body and have a low rating – 60 or under. Foods containing very few or no carbohydrates do not have a GI rating.

The ratings below are approximate. They can change depending on the product brand and your individual blood sugar level, which changes throughout the day. The GI values shown here are meant as a guideline to make better food choices.

Foods	GI Value	Foods	GI Value
Breads		**Breakfast Foods**	
Bagel	72	Buckwheat groats	45
Croissant	67	Cheerios	74
Muffin, English	70	Coco Puffs	80
Multi-grain	53	Cornflakes	81
Sprouted wheat	53	Corn Pops	80
Sourdough	54	Cream of wheat	66
White	70	French toast	67
Whole wheat	71	Fruit Loops	69
		Grits	69
Grains, cooked		Grapenuts	67
Amaranth	97	Kashi 7 Whole Grains	65
Barley	25	Museli	49
Basmati rice, white	57	Oatmeal, instant	58

Foods	GI Value	Foods	GI Value
Brown rice	55	Oatmeal, rolled	55
Bulgar	47	Pancakes, wheat	67
Couscous	65	Pancakes, buckwheat	100+
Millet	67	Raisin bran	61
Quinoa	53	Rice Krispies	82
Tortilla, corn	52	Rice Chex	89
Tortilla, flour	30	Special K	69
White rice	98	Total	76
Wild rice	57	Waffles	76
Pastas, cooked		**Vegetables**	
Brown rice noodles	92	Beets, raw	64
Buckwheat noodles	59	Carrots, raw	16
Macaroni, cooked	47	Carrots, cooked	47
Macaroni, whole wheat	37	Greens, cooked	32
Pasta, white flour	49	Peas, cooked	42
Udon noodles	55	Potato, white baked	72
White rice noodles	53	Potato, instant	87
Whole wheat noodles	37	Pumpkin, cooked	75
		Sweet corn, cooked	52
Fruits		Sweet potato, cooked	61
Apple	38	Tomatoes, cooked	38
Apricot	57	Winter squashes, cooked	75
Avocado	50	Yam, cooked	37
Banana	52	Most vegetables, cooked	32
Blueberries	40		

Eat Healthy. Be Healthy at Any Age.

Foods	GI Value	Foods	GI Value
Cantaloupe	65	**Juices and Soft Drinks**	
Cherries, sweet	22	Apple juice	41
Dates	42	Gatorade	89
Grapefruit	25	Cranberry juice	59
Grapes	46	Coca-Cola	63
Kiwi	53	Grapefruit juice	48
Mango	51	Orange juice	50
Orange	43	V8 juice	33
Papaya	59		
Peach	42	**Nuts and Seeds**	
Pear	38	Cashews	22
Pineapple	59	Mixed nuts	18
Raisins	64	Peanuts and peanut butter	14
Strawberries	55	Pecans	20
Watermelon	72	Sunflower seeds	20
		Walnuts	20
Beans and Lentils (cooked)			
Baked beans	48	**Dairy Products**	
Bean soup	64	Cheese, most	27
Black beans	20	Cow milk, whole	27
Chickpeas (garbanzos)	28	Cow milk, skim	32
Edamame (soy beans)	16	Ice cream, except choc.	61
Kidney beans	28	Rice milk	86
Lentils, brown	32	Soy milk	34
Lentils, red or green	26	Yogurt, plain	32
Lentil soup	44	Yogurt, low fat w/ fruit	31
Pinto beans	42		

Foods	GI Value	Foods	GI Value
Split pea soup	64	**Sweetners**	
White beans	13	Agave nectar	13
		Fructose	15
Snack Foods		Glucose	100+
Potato chips	56	Honey	61
Rice crackers	87	Sucrose	65
Popcorn	65		
Corn chips	74		

Sources: www.dietgrail.com/gid/ and www.glycemicindex.com/ foodSearch.php

APPENDIX 2

Foods for The Cleansing Program

Vegetables
Artichokes
Asparagus
Avocados
Bell peppers (all colors)
Beet greens
Broccoli
Brussels sprouts
Cabbage
Carrots (organic)
Celery
Cauliflower
Chard
Collard greens
Cucumber
Dandelion greens
Eggplant
Endive
Fennel
Garlic
Green beans
Green onions (scallions)
Kale
Kohlrabi
Leeks
Lettuces (all)
Mustard greens
Okra
Onions
Pea sprouts

Radishes
Snow or snap peas
Spinach
Sprouts
Squash, summer
String beans
Sunflower greens
Tomatoes
Turnip greens
Wheatgrass
Watercress
Zucchini

Other Things
Almonds
Chia seeds
Flax seeds
Hemp seeds
Coconuts
Grapefruit, white
Lemons
Limes

Water (with pH drops)
Distilled water
Reverse-osmosis
Purified
Selected bottled – Volvc,
  Voss, Essentia, Fiji

Herbs, Spices, and Seasonings
Cinnamon
Chili pepper
Cumin
Curry powde
Garlic
Ginger root
Herbs, organic (all)
Spice Hunter brand
  seasoning blends
Sea salt

Fats and Oils
Avocado oil, organic,
  extra virgin
Coconut oil, organic,
  extra virgin
Olive oil, organic, extra
  virgin

Milk
Coconut milk
Almond milk
Hemp seed milk

Foods Review

Healthy Foods

VEGETABLES
Artichokes
Asparagus
Barley grass
Bell peppers (all
  colors)
Beets
Beet greens
Broccoli
Brussels sprouts
Cabbage
Carrots (organic)
Celery
Cauliflower
Chard
Collard greens
Cucumber
Dandelion greens
Eggplant
Endive
Fennel
Garlic
Green beans
Green onions
  (scallions)
Jicama
Kale
Kohlrabi
Leeks
Lettuces (all)
Mustard greens
Okra
Onions

Parsnips
Peas (sweet, Eng-
  lish, snap)
Potatoes, red new
Radishes
Rutabagas
Seaweed (sea
  vegetables)
Snow peas
Spinach
Sprouts
Squash, summer
  and winter
String beans
Sunflower greens
Tomatoes
Turnip greens
Turnips
Wheatgrass
Watercress
Yams
Zucchini

**FRUITS (low
  sugar)**
Apples (when
  balanced)
Avocados
Blackberries
  (when balanced)
Blueberries
  (when balanced)

Boysenberries
  (when balanced)
Coconuts
Grapefruit
Lemons
Limes
Olives, green
  (no vinegar)
Pears (when
  balanced)
Raspberries
  (when balanced)
Strawberries
  (when balanced)

**BEANS and
  LEGUMES**
Adzuki
Black
Black-eyed
Cranberry
Garbanzo
Kidney
Lentils
Mung
Navy
Pinto
White

GRAINS
Amaranth
Basmati rice
  (brown)

Buckwheat
Flours (almond,
  spelt, millet,
  amaranth,
  kamut, quinoa)
Kamut
Millet
Quinoa
Spelt
Wild rice

WATER
Alkaline or
  Ionized
Distilled wa-
  ter (with pH
  drops)
Purified water
  (with pH drops)
Reverse-osmosis
  (with pH drops)

MILK
Coconut milk
Hemp seed milk
Nut and seed
  milks
Soy milk

**NUTS, SEEDS
and BUTTERS
(raw and
unsalted)**
Almonds and
  almond butter
  (raw)
Brazil nuts
Filberts
Flax seeds
Hemp seeds

Macadamia nuts
Pecans (when in
  season)
Pine nuts
Pumpkin seeds
Sesame seeds
Sunflower seeds
Tahini (sesame
  seed butter)
Walnuts (when in
  season)

**HERBS,
SPICES and
SEASONINGS**
Bragg® Liquid
  Aminos™
Cinnamon
Chili pepper
Cumin
Curry powder
Garlic
Ginger root
Herbs, organic
  (all)
Real Salt brand
  salt
Sea salt
Spice Hunter
  brand
  seasonings

FATS and OILS
Almond oil
Avocado oil
Borage oil
Coconut oil,
  organic, extra
  virgin
Flax seed oil

Grape seed oil
Hemp seed oil
Macadamia oil
Olive oil
Udo's Choice Oil
  Blend

**OTHER
PRODUCTS**
Boca Burgers
  (vegan)
Brown rice cakes
Edamame (fresh
  soybeans)
Fresh salsa (no
  vinegar)
Hummus
Manna bread
  (sun seed or
  whole wheat)
Oily fish – salm-
  on, trout (occa-
  sionally)
Pesto (vegan)
Rice noodles
Rotini
  noodles(quinoa
  or spelt)
Soba noodles
  (buckwheat)
Sprouted whole
  wheat tortillas
Stevia, Coconut
  crystals
Sun-dried toma-
  toes (in olive oil
  or sun dried)
Tofu
Vegetable broth
  (yeast free)

177

Eat Healthy. Be Healthy at Any Age.

Better Food Choices

From	To
Cow's milk	Almond, soy, rice, or hemp milk
Beef, chicken, pork, shellfish	Fresh wild salmon or trout (occasionally), Sprouted Organic Tofu
Cold cereal, oatmeal, pancakes	Millet, buckwheat, quinoa, cooked
Baked potato with butter	Basmati rice or red potato with olive oil
Coffee, soda, alcohol, fruit juice	Coconut water or alkaline water
1 quart of water each day	1 qt. of water for every 50 lbs. weight each day
Pizza, hamburger, fried chicken	Sprouted whole wheat tortilla wrap with veggies
Iceberg lettuce salad	Spinach/red leaf lettuce/ romaine with avocado
Vinegar or cream-based dressing	Olive oil-based dressing with lemon juice
Pasta with alfredo sauce	Buckwheat noodles with vegetables
Bread with jam	Brown rice cake or spelt cake with almond butter
Potato chips and ranch dip	Sprouted whole wheat tortilla chips with hummus or salsa
Candy, gum, cake, pie, donuts	Almonds, pumpkin seeds, raw veggies
Meat and starch meals	Vegetable and low-carbohydrate meals
Cooked or microwaved meals	Raw, steamed, or low-temperature meals
Sugar, artificial sweeteners	Stevia, Coconut crystals

List of Foods to Avoid

Alcohol	Fruits (sweet) – they feed
Animal products and by-	mycotoxins due to their sugar
products (except oily fish	Grains, stored and refined
occasionally)	Honey, agave, Sucanat, maple
Artificial sweeteners	syrup, sugar
Bread – unless no yeast;	Microwaved food
best sprouted	Most processed foods – they
Carob	are refined and contain added
Citric acids (fresh lemon ok)	chemicals
Cocoa	Mushrooms
Coffee	Oats
Corn	Peanuts
Dairy products, milk,	Pistachios
cheese, yogurt, butter, etc.	Potatoes, stored
Dried Fruit	Rye
Eggs	Vinegar
Fermented products	Wine – it is fermented

Do not buy products that contain added citric acid (a flavoring and preservative in foods and beverages), *mushrooms, yeast, vinegar, peanuts, or corn.* These products harbor mold, yeast, and fungus, or promote them in the body. These are called mycotoxins, and they resist being broken down during digestion. They remain in the food chain in meat and dairy products. Temperature treatments such as cooking and freezing do not destroy these toxins. They can result in disease, health problems, and weakened immune systems, and can manifest as allergens or irritants.

179

APPENDIX 4

Resource Guide

Supplements

The Cleansing Program Supplements
www.janefalke.com/store/cleansing-supplements/

Kitchen Equipment

Blenders, nut bags, Spirooli 3-in-1 Turning Slicer™, Saladacco Spiral Slicer™, dehydrator
www.rawgourmet.com
www.discountjuicers.com

Food processor – long-lasting food processors and other kitchen equipment
Costco
www.cuisinart.com

Canning jars
Most supermarkets

Food saver
Walmart

Debbie Meyer™ Green Bags®
Most supermarkets and natural food markets
www.debbiemeyer.com

Organic Produce and Dried Food Distributors

Fresh, organically grown fruits, vegetables, and dried foods delivered to your door
www.diamondorganics.com

High-quality organic dried food distributors
www.sunorganicfarm.com

Organic sprouted tofu, super firm, plain
  natural food markets
  www.wildwoodfoods.com

Organic herbs and spices
  www.spicehunter.com
  www.frontiercoop.com
  www.sunorganicfarms.com

Mauk Family Farms Raw Mineral Rich Crusts™
  natural food markets
  www.maukfamilyfarms.com, 714-547-7977

Suzie's Spelt Puffed Cakes™ (regular flavor)
  www.goodgroceries.com

*Edward & Sons Organic Creamed Coconut™ and
100% Organic Coconut Flakes*
  natural food markets
  www.edwardandsons.com

Coconut Secret Raw Coconut Crystals™ (organic)
  natural food markets
  www.coconutsecret.com 888-369-3393

Lydia's Organics Sprouted Cinnamon Cereal™
  natural food markets
  www.lydiasorganics.com

Herbamare® Original organic seasoning salt
  Most supermarkets and natural food markets
  www.herbamare.us

*Spice Hunter's The Zip®, Mild Blend, all-purpose
seasoning*
  www.spicehunter.com

Vegan Recipes
  www.nutritionmd.org/recipes/index.html

Eat Healthy. Be Healthy at Any Age.

Type in food you want to use. Many recipes pop up.

Tools for Health

A body mass index (BMI) calculator is an easy-to-use tool for estimating your body fat using your weight and height.
www.nhlbisupport.com/bmi/

Track meals and count calories
http://hp2010.nhlbihin.net/menuplanner/menu.cgi

Science

Learn about tropical oils at www.coconutoil.com

Magazines, Articles, and Communities

Articles about healthy living
www.healthfree.com

Articles and recipes about healthy living
www.naturalhealthmag.com
www.alkalinesisters.com

Alternative Health Education Centers and Programs

A comprehensive program where you can learn The Living Foods Lifestyle®
www.annwigmore.org

Natural and alternative health care and education
www.hippocratesinst.org

An intense three-week internal cleansing program and healing modality
www.optimumhealth.org

A holistic medical spa where you can learn the raw food lifestyle
www.treeoflife.nu

Nutrition and detoxification with doctor-assisted medical care
www.sanoviv.com

Notes by Chapter

Chapter 2 – Change Your Health By Changing Your Eating

1. *60 Minutes*, "Flavorists," (November 27, 2011 and September 2, 2012)
2. www.truthinlabeling.org, ingredients names used to hide MSG in food, retrieved 6/21/2011.
3. John E. Erb and T. Michelle Erb, *The Slow Poisoning of America*, (Paladins Press, Virginia Beach, Virginia, 2003) p.105.

Chapter 3 – Who Controls Our Food?

1. Ronnie Cummins and Ben Lilliston, *Genetically Engineered Food: A Self-Defense Guide for Consumers*, (Marlow & Company, New York, 2004) p. 15.
2. http://en.wikipedia.org/wiki/Genetically_modified_food, retrieved February 8, 2009.
3. Staff, "Genetically Modified (GM) Food: A Guide for the Confused", (August 29, 2006) retrieved September 8, 2006, from www.organicconsumers.org/2006/article._1860.cfm, (p. 3).
4. Cummins and Lilliston, *Genetically Engineered Food* pp. 103, 106, 107, 108.
5. Jeffrey M. Smith, *Seeds of Deception: Exposing Industry and Government Lies about the Safety of the Genetically Engineered Foods You're Eating,* (Chelsea Green Publishing, White River Junction, VT, 2003) p. 157.
6. ibid., p. 236.
7. Mayo Clinic Staff, "Organic foods: Are they safer? More nutritious?" (2006, December 20) Retrieved October 11, 2007, from www.mayoclinic.com/health/organic-food/NU00255
8. www.ewg.org/foodnews/list/ retrieved 4/25/12
9. Morgan Spurlock, *Super Size Me: A Film of Epic Portions*, 2004.

10. Marion Nestle, interview, "How the Food Industry Influences What We Eat," *Nutrition Action Health Letter*, Center for Science in the Public Interest, (October 2011).

11. T. Colin Campbell and Thomas M. Campbell II, *The China Study: Startling Implications for Diet, Weight Loss and Long-term Health.* (BenBella Books, Dallas, TX, 2005) p. 249.

Chapter 4 – Carbohydrates: The Body's Fuel

1. Mary G. Enig, *Know Your Fats: The Complete Primer for Understanding the Nutrition of Fats, Oils and Cholesterol,* (Bethesda Press, Silver Spring, MD, 2000) p. 56.

Chapter 5 – Fats: The Real Truth

1. Elson M. Haas, *Staying Healthy with Nutrition: The Complete Guide to Diet and Nutitional Medicine,* (Celestial Arts, Berkeley, CA, 2006) p. 73.

2. F. Davidson, et. al., "Cholesterol, coconuts, and diet on Polynesian atolls: a natural experiment: the Pukapuka and Tokelau island studies." *American Journal of Clinical Nutrition*, 1981 Aug; 34(8):1552-61.

Chapter 6 – Protein: The Treasured Nutrient

1. L. A. Frassetto et al, "Worldwide Incidence of Hip Fracture in Elderly Women: Relation to Consumption of Animal and Vegetable Foods", *Gerontology* Vol. 55 (2000): M585-M592.

2. Ronald F. Schmid, *Traditional Foods Are Your Best Medicine: Improving Health and Longevity with Native Nutrition.*(Healing Arts Press, Rochester, VT, 1997) p. 160-161.

3. T. Colin Campbell and Thomas M. Campbell II, *The China Study: Startling Implications for Diet, Weight Loss and Long-term Health.*(BenBella Books, Dallas, TX, 2005).

4. "Dietary Reference Intakes for Energy, Carbohydrate,

Eat Healthy. Be Healthy at Any Age.

Fiber, Fat, Fatty Acids, Cholesterol, Protein, and Amino Acids", Institute of Medicine of National Academies, (September 5, 2002) retrieved 1/31/2012 from www.iom.edu/Reports/2002/Dietary-Reference-Intakes-for-Energy-Carbohydrate-Fiber-Fat-Fatty-Acids-Cholesterol-Protein-and-Amino-Acids.aspx#

5. B. Farmer et al, "A Vegetarian Dietary Pattern as a Nutrient-Dense Approach to Weight Management: An Analysis of the National Health and Nutrition Examination Survey 1999-2004", formerly the Journal of the American Dietetic Association, June 2011; 111, Issue 6, Pages 819-827. www.journals.elsevierhealth.com/periodicals/yjada/article/S0002-8223(11)00275-6/abstract

Chapter 7 – Micronutrients: The Workhorses of Health

1. L. Packer and C. Colman, *The Antioxidant Miracle: Put Lipoic acid, Pycnogenol, and Vitamins E and C to Work for You*, (Wiley & Sons, New York, 2000) p. 32.

Chapter 8 – Non-Nutrients: Essential to Health

1. Otto Warburg, lecture, "The Prime Cause and Prevention of Cancer", June 30, 1966, http://healingtools.tripod.com/primecause1.html/ retrieved 1/31/2012.

Chapter 9 – A Chance for Change

• Most of the information in this chapter comes from The Awareness Game™ poster and the Playing by the Rules of Life workshop (copyright 1995) developed by Pete Wanger and Jane Wanger-Falke.

Chapter 10 – Benefits of Regular Exercise

• Much of the information used to write this chapter came from the Patient Education

Institute, Inc. at www.nlm.nih.gov/medlineplus/
tutorials/exercisingforahealthylife/htm/_no_50_
no_0.htm retrieved 3/12/12

- For more support and information about exercise
go to www.healthfinder.gov. There is a physical
activity tracker and food tracker to help you with
your weekly goals.

Chapter 11 – Why Cleanse the Internal Body?

- The source of the photos in this chapter is from -
The Microscopy Course materials, 2010.

Chapter 15 – The Maintenance Program

1. Microscopy course taken by Jane Falke - June and
September 2010.

About the Jane Falke

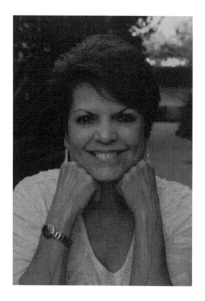

While growing up, Jane didn't have a burning desire to change the world or make a difference. She was taught to get married and raise children. Within a few years of being married at age 19, Jane had two children within eleven months. She was doing what she was taught to do, take care of children, a husband, a house and yard and worked a full time job in real estate loans and sales.

Jane's daughter had type 1 diabetes at the age of two. Learning to balance her diet and giving insulin injections was of utmost importance in keeping her daughter alive. She learned that measuring three main foods, carbohydrates, proteins and fats, would keep her daughter balanced and avoid a diabetic reaction or coma. This was when food sparked an interest in Jane. Nutrition wasn't even a word Jane knew or understood at that time. However, she realized that balancing a diet was important to maintain health.

After the children were grown, Jane's husband was diagnosed with cancer. His poor eating habits were a clue to his disease. Six months later he past away. That was when Jane decided to explore nutrition as a possible cause of many of the diseases in our society today.

During the next 20 years Jane studied food and nutrition from a natural prospective. She now holds a Masters degree in Holistic Nutrition. She has an Associate Chef and Instructor certification and The Science of Raw Food Nutrition certification from the Living Light Culinary Arts Institute. She is certified in Plant-Based Nutrition from eCornell and T. Colin Campbell Foundation, and has been a certified yoga teacher since 1991. In 2010, Jane was trained by Dr. Robert O. Young in live and dry blood analysis, a method that offers a way clients can see the condition of their blood and make dietary changes to correct imbalances and help prevent disease.

As a Holistic Nutritionist, Jane considers the whole being both body and mind. She educates and inspires clients to *remove the cause of their symptoms*, not to look for a magic pill that may only reduce or temporarily remove symptoms. Through nutritional changes and live and dry blood analysis, Jane has seen in her clients early symptoms of major diseases and has helped to change the cause of these symptoms by teaching a natural way of eating by balancing the body's nutritional needs. She shares her knowledge so people will make better choices and change what they eat, drink and think.

Jane works with clients who are tired, sluggish, overweight, stressed and unhappy with their chronic conditions and want to take control of their health through a plant-based diet, balanced nutrition, and lifestyle change.

At this writing, Jane is 71 years old. She eats a natural, mostly plant-based diet and is physically and mentally healthy without the need of daily medications like most of her clients. She has practiced yoga and meditation for over 20 years and feeling her lifestyle has contributed to her good health.

Eat Healthy. Be Healthy at Any Age.

Jane is the Founder of The Nutritionist Naturally with a mission to provide products and services that educate and inspire people about food and nutrition so they can maintain a long and healthy life.

For more information about Jane and her life-changing work, visit www.JaneFalke.com

Made in the USA
San Bernardino, CA
08 April 2014